EATING ANXIETY

EATING ANXIETY

The Perils of Food Politics

CHAD LAVIN

University of Minnesota Press

Minneapolis

London

A version of chapter 5 was published previously as Chad Lavin, "The Year of Eating Politically," *Theory & Event* 12, no. 2 (2009); copyright 2009 by Chad Lavin and The Johns Hopkins University Press; reprinted with permission by The Johns Hopkins University Press. Portions of chapter 6 appeared in Chad Lavin, "The Vegetarian Lesson," *The Chronicle Review (The Chronicle of Higher Education)*, August 14, 2011.

Published by the University of Minnesota Press
111 Third Avenue South, Suite 290
Minneapolis, MN 55401-2520
http://www.upress.umn.edu

Library of Congress Cataloging-in-Publication Data
Lavin, Chad.
   Eating anxiety : the perils of food politics / Chad Lavin.
   Includes bibliographical references and index.
   ISBN 978-0-8166-8091-7 (hc : alk. paper) — ISBN 978-0-8166-8092-4 (pb : alk. paper)
   1. Diet—Political aspects—United States.   2. Food industry and trade—Political aspects—United States.   I. Title.
   TX360.U6L38 2013
   338.1'9—dc23   2012048338

Printed in the United States of America on acid-free paper

The University of Minnesota is an equal-opportunity educator and employer.

20   19   18   17   16   15   14   13   10   9   8   7   6   5   4   3   2   1

CONTENTS

ACKNOWLEDGMENTS

I started writing this book in the fall of 2005, soon after a hurricane and a shameful display of political neglect sent me fleeing from Louisiana to Texas to Pennsylvania, fortunate enough to find helpful friends, family, and strangers at each step along the way. I finished writing six years later, five days before the birth of my son. These events do more than bookend the writing of this book. They each, in their own way, capture the exposure and intimacy that are rarely avoidable in considerations of food and politics and that are at the center of this project. In fleeing a flooded city (an experience of fear and outrage punctuated by great moments of compassion) and witnessing the birth of my own child (an experience of joy and wonder marked with tremendous anxiety), I found myself experiencing similar feelings of vulnerability and gratitude that come, invariably, from the sharing of spaces, ideas, tragedies, and opportunities with others. Digesting such experiences—as well as countless other more prosaic events—would be impossible without the material and psychological sustenance provided by people and institutions daily and as a matter of course.

This book was nourished in similar but more immediate and obvious ways by the various people and communities who read, solicited, listened to, or commented directly on its contents. Individually, these people include Asma Abbas, Rebecca Bamford, Mark Barrow, Ryan Carey, Bill Chaloupka, Kevin Corrigan, Jodi Dean, Kennan Ferguson, Johnnie Goldfinger, Jim Klagge, Mike Lipscomb, Nancy Love, Tim Luke, Brad MacDonald, Elizabeth Mazzolini, Wolfgang Natter, Amy Nelson, Paul Passavant, Lydia Patton, Joe Pitt, Andrew Radde-Gallwitz, Chris Russill, Holloway Sparks, Maryann Tebben, Katie Terezakis, Larry Torcello, Shane Vogel, Deborah White, and Kathryn Wichelns. They also include the students in my classes on food at Emory University, Hobart and William Smith Colleges, and Virginia Tech. These folks were all kind enough to indulge my often frustrating engagements with this material, and they somehow managed to inject their own critical approaches into my own occasionally imperious readings. Pieter Martin at the University of Minnesota Press shepherded this manuscript through the various hurdles of academic publishing and offered some very thoughtful last-minute suggestions for revision. The book is surely better because of each of their contributions. (I have to think I am as well.)

Great thanks go to Martine Watson Brownley, as well as the wonderful staff and my fellow fellows at the Bill and Carol Fox Center for Humanistic Inquiry at Emory University for generously hosting (and feeding) me during the 2006–7 school year. This project never would have proceeded past the first chapter without both the moral and material support I received while there. The College of Liberal Arts and Human Sciences at Virginia Tech later came through with another welcome grant to help me finish the project in the summer of 2011. Thanks to the division of Social Sciences of Bard College at Simon's Rock, the departments of Political Science and Environmental Studies at Winthrop University, and the department of Philosophy at the Rochester Institute of Technology for inviting me to talk through some of these issues as I worked on them. Additional thanks to the departments of Political Science at Hobart and William Smith Colleges and Virginia Tech and to my colleagues in the ASPECT program at Virginia Tech for providing welcome and inspiring places to live, work, and write.

But it is surely to Elizabeth, my true companion, whose life has intersected with mine in ways too wonderful to state, whose critical eye has greatly improved how I write and think, who pointed me toward food politics then provided both focused and casual remarks that improved every part of this book (even the parts that continue to irritate her), and whose love, humor, and strength helped me endure too many years of commuting up and down the Eastern Seaboard, that I owe the most. And to Walter, who somehow manages a smile as breathtaking as his mother's. Here's to never eating alone.

INTRODUCTION

Food Politics in the Twilight of Sovereignty

IN RECENT YEARS, FOOD HAS emerged as one of the more pervasive issues in political struggle, popular entertainment, and humanist scholarship. Politically, the media warns of a global food crisis owing to rapidly rising prices and drought-induced shortages, even as the developed world faces a mounting public health threat stemming from widespread *over*eating and continues to redirect so much grain toward biofuel production. On television, contenders for *Iron Chef* or *Top Chef* delight audiences with their spectacular meals and culinary skill, while the contestants on *The Biggest Loser* remind the audiences of the perils of indulgence. Academically, the growing interest in "food studies" wrangles anthropologists, historians, philosophers, and nutritionists together to reveal the hidden machinations of an exploitative, inequitable, and unsustainable global food system while also celebrating the opportunities for human expression and joy through cultural rites and regional identity. In each case, with a precious and tempting resource implicated in discourses of personal identity, global inequality, and cultural authenticity, food appears as paradoxically both fascinating and frightening. *Eating Anxiety*, as a work of political theory, situates each of these factors, and each of these issues, in a historical condition anxious about the meaning of and possibilities for human freedom. The aim of this study is, therefore, threefold: first, to explain how food functions culturally, politically, and metaphorically to help structure popular and philosophical understandings of the world and the place of humans within it; second, to introduce the concept of "digestive subjectivity" and show how it offers valuable resources for rethinking cherished political ideals surrounding knowledge, identity, and power; and third, to unpack some of the debates in contemporary food politics, showing how digestive subjectivity offers critical resources for navigating contemporary political crises over globalization, neoliberalism, and democracy.

While the vegetarianism and food co-ops of an earlier era may have been dismissed as alternative lifestyles or fashion statements, today the case hardly needs to be made that food is a political issue. Arguments about everything from industrial pesticides to agricultural subsidies to dietary regulation circulate freely in Whole Foods and Wal-Mart, schools and churches, Congress and the UN. This could be because our current global food system—consuming so much water and oil and producing so much sewage and carbon dioxide—is unavoidably implicated in ongoing and impending economic and ecological crises. But it is surely also because, as Elspeth Probyn notes, considerations of food inevitably blur boundaries between discrete lines of thought and areas of study, as studying the production, distribution, and consumption of food necessarily forces attention to the science of diet; the ethics of animal husbandry; the economics of land distribution; and the sociology of class, culture, and taste.[1] Indeed, medical investigations into nutrition readily lead to questions about marketing; the work of agricultural engineers has bearing on demography and migration patterns; and anthropological work on cuisine cannot be disentangled from questions of global trade, animal welfare, and industrial subsidies. Food, in other words, is rarely only food.

The popularity of food politics might owe to another issue. When we eat, our bodies fuse with—and become momentarily indistinguishable from—the world that surrounds us. Objects that were once part of the external world are literally in*corporate*d into the self, and the space that separates the self from the world is collapsed. Michael Pollan, perhaps the era's most visible food writer and the current face of food politics, draws on this realization when he states at the opening of his best seller, *The Omnivore's Dilemma*, that "the way we eat represents our most profound engagement with the natural world."[2] This intimacy—this moment of allowing the natural world to invade the bounded space of our bodies, to enter into our mouths and then biochemically become part of the self—amounts to an experience of the limits of the self. This moment of considering and confounding the border between *me* and *not me* offers a singular opportunity for examining understandings of identity, authenticity, and responsibility that form the backbone of contemporary political ideologies. As a result, I contend, trends in food politics often have their stakes not in the production and distribution of food, nor even in abstract commitments to equality, but rather in the integrity of the border that supposedly separates the self from the world that remains an axiomatic requirement of personal identity. Further, because discourses of ethics, aesthetics, ecology, and politics all consider how or why we can or should violate this border—how or why we can or should engage, appropriate, or surrender to the forces that confront us—I argue that this singular experience of this border in the physical act of eating offers a distilled and intensified terrain for thinking about the more generalized questions of ethics, aesthetics, ecology, and politics.

When famed agrarian philosopher Wendell Berry states, in a now often repeated statement, that "eating is an agricultural act," he calls attention to how food blurs another border: that between public and private.[3] In Berry's formulation, choices made in the home have profound impact on the organization of space and resources in a society, helping to determine how, where, and which foods will be produced and, thus, how resources like water and land will be allocated and used. This argument, echoed in popular works from Michael Pollan, Eric Schlosser, and Barbara Kingsolver, has sent ever more consumers to farmers' markets in the belief that their shopping habits can produce a different, more sustainable system of agriculture.[4] In this now popular idea about rebuilding food culture through responsible consumption, what happens at the dinner table (a space as charged as any other with the sentiments of the private sphere and individual choice) becomes paradigmatically public, essential to understanding the distribution of resources and opportunities in an industrial society.

As another example of the ability of food to challenge cherished borders, note the popular discourse of animal rights that animates so much vegetarian literature. Animal rights advocates have long defended themselves against a presumed reductionism by arguing that extending the discourse of rights does not require treating animals as if they were human. That is, we need not give cows the vote. But in doing so, they tend to ignore a larger contradiction in their position. The discourse of legal rights is predicated on the ideal of sovereign, rational beings being afforded protections and opportunities equal to that of others; it applies an abstract principle to a population of abstracted and selfsame individuals. The discourse of *animal* rights, however, rejects this notion of an abstract or universal subject that underwrites the humanism that itself legitimates the discourse of rights. In other words, animal rights attempts to mobilize a humanist conceit toward posthumanist ends, disregarding the fact that by calling into question the discourse of humanism they also call into question the discourse of species that explains *why* certain beings deserve protection to begin with. Today, when biomedicine and biotechnology are similarly giving lie to the conceits of humanism, discourses of vegetarianism capitalize on a growing anxiety about this conceptual border that still proves indispensable to agriculture and contemporary political affairs.

Eating Anxiety examines these borders—between self and world, between public and private, and between human and nonhuman—and explores how the singular experience of eating affords a concentrated moment for reckoning with how such conceptual and institutional borders organize our lives. These challenges prove especially salient today, as the nature of global political order is similarly called into question due to the challenge of another set of cherished borders: the territorial borders that separate discrete and governable states. These challenges to those territorial borders by flows of bodies, information, and capital are typically grouped under the banner of "globalization," and what they mean for the prospects of global order has grown into one of the more pressing political questions of our era. This book reads these different kinds of border violations side by side, and argues that the violations of the borders of the self in the physical act of eating offers a metonymically intensified version of the collapse of territorial borders by the forces of globalization. The book thus identifies in the contemporary condition a matched set of crises, as the assumptions underlying both individual sovereignty and national sovereignty come under fire from technological, political, and philosophical developments of the past few decades.

The premise of the current project is that the dominant political debates of recent years—from those surrounding globalization and terrorism to those over the meaning of abortion and individual responsibility—can all be traced to a disruption in the various borders that have organized political thinking. *Eating Anxiety* uses the occasion of food to visit the threats to and the sustainability of borders—most notably the borders of the individual, the species, and the nation-state—that have organized political, ethical, aesthetic, and scientific discourses for centuries. More specifically, I argue that food, as the artifact that most visibly reveals the tenuousness of the ontological assumptions of liberal political thought, is a ready artifact for both displacing and examining those disruptions. In other words, beneath the medical veneer of the debates about obesity we can find widespread anxieties about the status of the narrative of individual responsibility that anchors liberal politics. Scratching the surface of debates about vegetarianism reveals an underlying anxiety not about how we treat animals but about the tenability of taxonomic demarcations that justify our approach to both rights and property. Behind the exhortation to "eat local" stands a pronounced anxiety about the meaning of lived space and the possibility of representative democracy in an era of globalization.

That we approach food with anxiety is something of an axiom for this project. This anxiety is on clear display in any number of approaches to food and food politics. Television shows like *The Biggest Loser*, documentary films like *Super Size Me* and *Food, Inc*, and vegetarian manifestos like *Animal Liberation* call attention to how our food habits pose a threat to ourselves and others. Books with titles like *Fat Land, Safe Food, Stuffed and Starved*, and *The Food Wars* sound blaring alarms about the organization of agriculture and food under globalization,[5] while *Big Fat Lies, Food Fight, Food Politics*, and *The Omnivore's Dilemma* appeal to concerns that consumers do not (or cannot) know what is in their food, that dietary advice is dominated by a multibillion-dollar diet industry, or that the organic labeling process and food regulation more broadly are irretrievably corrupt.[6] Even daily conversations about food rarely avoid the many threats posed by the American diet, with mentions of trans fats, high-fructose corn syrup, and salmonella seemingly overshadowing more relaxed consideration of taste, pleasure, or even nourishment. I argue that the saturation of food discourse with fear and anxiety is symptomatic of broader concerns about economic power, self-determination, and the reliability of government institutions and the scientific establishment. Most generally, *Eating Anxiety* argues that the dynamics of contemporary food politics consolidate and intensify the same concerns about individual safety and political powerlessness on display in the rise of gated communities, market fetishism, border vigilantism, and support for an increasingly punitive criminal justice system.

At the same time, my argument cannot be reduced to a claim that diffuse and unwieldy political anxieties are displaced onto food. Rather, and as we shall see, discourses of food also participate in a novel technology of population management in which, as Foucault puts it, "life and its mechanisms [are brought] into the realm of explicit calculations and . . . knowledge-power [is made] an agent of transformation of human life."[7] In his lectures on what he calls "biopolitics," Foucault explicitly links this technology to liberal reforms of limited, representative government and capitalist markets,[8] and, indeed, the discourses of food at the opening of the twenty-first century participate in a trend toward property rights, individual responsibility, heightened surveillance, and data collection that is essential to neoliberal order. This is true not only in the discourse of diet and exercise—where individuals assume responsibility for self-discipline by tracking what they eat, what they do, and how quickly they move[9]—but also in technologies of surveillance and data management that are mobilized to battle the current "epidemic" of obesity, and the popular vegetarian cry that the torture of animals and exploitation of workers in American slaughterhouses is best remedied through the market mechanism of individual consumers boycotting the meat industry. In other words, social order is achieved not through hierarchical and top-down authoritative rules but through bottom-up technologies of individual responsibility and voluntary participation.

The linkage of food politics to neoliberalism can be seen in the work of the high priest of responsible foods, Michael Pollan. Giving voice to a common sentiment, Pollan declares that Americans are interested in taking control of their food—as evidenced by the rising interest in farmers' markets, backyard gardening, and localism—because "so much about life in a global economy feels as though it has passed beyond the individual's control."[10] There are a number of points to emphasize about Pollan's diagnosis: that he confirms what I am calling the anxieties of globalization, identifying a concern about powerlessness as endemic to our current era; that he offers food politics as a means to offset rather than confront those anxieties; and that the consumerist solutions he ultimately promotes in his widely read book appeal to a population increasingly disenchanted with or cynical about more conventionally political solutions to political problems. But more generally, Pollan's ideas about responsible consumerism promote classically liberal ideals of self-reliance and self-governance in a manner that resonates with the neoliberal trend toward market supremacy and individual responsibility. Like so much moral condemnation of the overweight for lacking self-control, advocates of responsible consumerism like Pollan and others promoting the purchase of organic, local, or sustainable food enact the biopolitical demand for self-governance and establish the market as the site of political change. They shift, in other words, the location of politics from the public to the private sphere, from the state to the market, more or less in lockstep with the political apparatus of neoliberalism. Far from a challenge to the forces of the global economy that allow so many to feel as though their life is beyond their control, such responses often contribute to them.[11]

Eating and Identity

The paradox of food being both fascinating and frightening probably owes to another paradox: that it both enables us to be what we are (by keeping us alive) and it changes what we are (by blurring the line that separates the self from the world). This paradox finds expression in some of the earliest and most enduring narratives of food that we know. How could we forget, after all, that it is Adam's act of eating that both keeps him alive and makes us mortal? More immediately, this is precisely why sharing food remains the centerpiece of so many religious festivals; the ritual consumption of the same material substance both celebrates and consecrates political and ethical community.[12] Among anthropologists and sociologists, the role food plays in solidifying local, regional, and national cultures reveals how identity is not achieved through heroic expressions of individuation but rather through passive internalization of social mores. More materially, this same paradox is expressed in the folk wisdom that "you are what you eat," an expression that conveys how we are simultaneously distinct from (*you* are) and entirely the same as that which surround us (*what* you eat).

How to feel about this paradoxical relationship to food, in fact, defines some of the dominant cleavages in the history of political thought. Leon Kass, for instance, indicts the mantra "you are what you eat" on principle for reducing humanity to raw matter and denying the dignity of the human form.[13] Such a materialist approach, he argues, justifies any number of violent and abominable pursuits, treating humans as just so much matter to be manipulated, essentially indistinguishable from the animals and vegetables that are rightly human food. Without reference to something that transcends embodiment (for Kass, a soul), one lacks a justification for eating carrots and cows but refusing to eat other human bodies. For Kass, we are not *what* we eat, but *how* we eat. Contrast this with another philosopher prone to use the experience of eating to help understand what it means to be a human being: Friedrich Nietzsche. In *Ecce Homo* and *On the Genealogy of Morals*, Nietzsche declares that one "becomes who one is" not by defining oneself against—but rather by experiencing a vulnerability to—the world.[14] While "a strong and well-constituted man digests his experiences (his deeds and misdeeds included) as he digests his meals,"[15] Nietzsche diagnoses two kinds of "sick animals" that lack such a constitution: the ascetic priest who "treats life as a wrong road" and is committed to "floating above life rather than in repose," and the man of *ressentiment* who is "a dyspeptic—he cannot 'have done' with anything."[16] For Nietzsche, both of these animals—suffering from anorexia and indigestion, respectively—miss that we are *because* we eat. A third approach to eating and identity can be found in Karl Marx, who approaches the issue of digestion more obliquely, using the language of food to structure what he takes to be the fundamental human activity: labor. Describing both labor and commerce as "social metabolism,"[17] Marx suggests that economic activity and digestive activity amount to the same process: mixing of self with world in a thermodynamic transfer of energy. In this dialectical approach, we are not only what we eat but also what eats us.

Each of these approaches to food will be explored in more detail in the chapters that follow. But for now note that even as Kass breaks radically from the materialisms of Nietzsche and Marx with his Platonic emphasis on the importance of an eternal human form, he shares with them a metaphorical treatment of eating, such that the way in which we encounter and assimilate the world informs not just a biological treatment of resources and metabolism but intensified discourses of ethics and identity that are essential to the constitution of self. In each, we can understand the central animating principle of human life—whether it is soul (Kass), will (Nietzsche), or value (Marx)—through food. Exploiting these metaphorics through this book, I will argue for a discourse of human and nonhuman life through the terms of eating and explore the political implications of what I call the digestive subject, which stands in contrast to a more common figure in liberal political thought: the sovereign subject.

My premise throughout this book is that food operates as a seductive metaphor for so many aspects of the human condition *not* because of food's singular position in the maintenance of human life but rather because the paradoxes that are made so visible in the act of eating are familiar from other domains of life. Another way to say this—one that I will repeat throughout the book—is that discourses of food are often not about food at all but about a more general existential condition in which individual identity is threatened by encounters and violations from a supposedly external world. Digestion, that is, often functions as what George Lakoff and Mark Johnson call a "structural metaphor" in which the specific characteristics of the activity of consumption are allowed to stand in for a more general "existential gestalt."[18]

This premise might seem unremarkable, but its implications are significant. I aim to argue that current organizations of power and information threaten a particular conception of subjectivity that serves as the foundation for dominant understandings of politics. In particular, I argue that for the past four centuries, the notion of individual sovereignty, itself predicated on an ontological and epistemological presumption of discretely bounded and autonomous subjects, has formed the philosophical foundations for global order based on limited, representative government and the authority of scientific truth. The presumed separation of subjects and objects underwrites not only commonsense ideas about scientific objectivity and personal identity but also established arguments for the legitimacy of property rights and political representation. A breakdown of this ideal—a breakdown displayed earlier in Kass, Nietzsche, and Marx and described with my term "digestive subjectivity"—provokes what Bruno Latour has identified as a "crisis of objectivity" that threatens established ideas about meaning, responsibility, and democracy.[19]

In a sense, this argument is nothing new. Marxists, feminists, and communitarians have been attacking a fetishized notion of individual identity for decades. More recently, political theorists such as Stephen White and William Connolly have sought to reveal how ontologies—ideas about the nature of being—necessarily underwrite political understandings. For White, questions of ontology are "entangled with questions of identity and history, with how we articulate the meaning of our lives, both individually and collectively."[20] Connolly offers the neologism "ontopolitical" to capture how particular ideas about the nature of bodies and force "fix possibilities, distribute explanatory elements, generate parameters within which an ethic is generated, and center (or decenter) assessments of identity, legitimacy, and responsibility."[21] While critical studies of the body from philosophers and anthropologists have tried to reveal how and why the notion of an invulnerable and coherent body became useful to a particular way of organizing political life,[22] a recent work titled *New Materialisms* endeavors to show how scientific and theoretical developments in physics and ontology through the twentieth century suggest renewed "reflection upon who or what should be taken as subjects and objects of ethical, legal, or political action."[23]

But again, my thesis is not that food has become an artifact of fascination because it is unique but precisely because it is generalizable. With the flourishing of biotechnology and cybernetics, the integrity of the individual body and the distinction of the human species have become increasingly untenable. As a direct result, the field of bioethics has developed to help guide medical and scientific practice through an increasingly hazy set of borders that are called on to bear the weight of important decisions. The most notable of these borders are those between alive and dead and human and nonhuman, and the blurring of these borders has provoked a series of controversies surrounding routine decisions about terminal and prenatal care, with passionate disagreement about when life begins and ends, and what sorts of organisms deserve the protections that come with being called human. Beyond this, however, practices formerly the purview of science fiction but now squarely within the domain of corporate scientific research to manufacture living tissue—for human organ transplants or for food—raise not only ethical questions about the manipulation of life and the treatment of animals but also existential questions about life, identity, and humanity.[24] Debates about teaching Darwin in schools or the moral status of embryonic stem cells, just like the metabolic conversion of a cow's muscle tissue into a part of my body, turn on questions (and anxieties) about the status of the self, what it means to be a human being, and how we ought to be in the world.

The stakes here are in a particular conception of identity and humanity that underwrites most everything we know about property, ethics, epistemology, and politics. The ideal of a discrete and bounded subject—sovereign over itself and separable from the world that surrounds it—underwrites dominant ideas about property, responsibility, objectivity, and representation. My claim in this book is that the rhetoric and experience of digestion disrupts this, and a fascination with that disruption corresponds to a real threat to the institutions and ideals that legitimate liberal governance. By exploring the terms and implications of this digestive approach to subjectivity, *Eating Anxiety* promises novel interpretations of some important texts from the canon of political theory, and thus a reworked mechanism by which to examine the relationship of identity and politics. The book, in other words, promises insight not just into food politics but into how understandings of food structure the very possibility of politics.

Privatizing Food

One of the great opportunities afforded by food for understanding politics is that it freely and regularly transgresses the border that supposedly separates the public and the private. Eating, again, has long played a central role in defining cultures by establishing shared conventions, tastes, rituals, and traditions; the material and cultural ritual of "breaking bread" serves in the production and consecration of community by ritualizing our shared constitution by the same material substance. This reconciliation of the individual and the community finds its most literal expression in the taking of Holy Communion. But it is also on display in more prosaic realms: from the ubiquitous claims that farmer's markets "build community" to the now familiar claim that the restaurant, as a site of urban sociality invented in eighteenth-century Paris, proved indispensable to the French revolutionary spirit.[25] Communal eating, in other words, merges the traditionally public and the traditionally private, consummating and restoring the bonds of ethical and political life. Just consult the *Oxford English Dictionary*:

> Consummate, "to add up, make up, to bring to an end, finish off, to complete, finish, to achieve, accomplish, to perfect. . . . Compare earlier . . . C O N S U M E "[26]

> Restore, from "Middle French *restorer* . . . to bring (a person or part of a person's body) back to health . . . Compare later R E S T A U R " (cf., restaurant).[27]

And yet in the contemporary United States, food is almost invariably couched in the rhetoric of individual choice and taste, with our decisions about food ("I don't like tomatoes" or "I'm a vegetarian") standing alongside decisions about lifestyle and sexuality as expressions of individual identity. Since World War II, cultural critics have pointed to the privatization of food in the United States as part of their lamentations of lost community. Prior to the 1950s, the argument goes, preparing meals required a significant amount of domestic labor, which practically compelled families to eat together. But developments in the production, processing, and packaging of food or fast food—from Cheez Whiz to the Happy Meal—have all but eliminated the need for collective eating. As a result, Americans eat more meals in their cars and fewer with their families. With the decline in family meals being a symbolic front in the ongoing cultural wars, concerns about alienation, exploitation, family values, and civic engagement that have occupied theorists and pundits for decades are regularly couched in the rhetorics and politics of food.[28]

The paradox is thus clear: typically couched in the individualistic language of individual choice and taste, how we eat is determined in large part by economic development and is a common lever in the cultural politics of race, gender, and the family. This is probably most clear when we recognize how the fretting over the decline in family meals is inseparable from the politics of feminism, as developments in food technology allowed so many women, formerly occupied with the arduous task of feeding a family, the freedom necessary to enter the paid labor force. While previous decades found "working moms" indicted in attempts to explain rising rates of crime and teen pregnancy, now the lack of "home cooking" is regularly pointed to as a primary cause of childhood obesity. Even as the politics of obesity remain grounded in the rhetorics of individual responsibility and self-governance, the *causes* of obesity are typically linked to the changing lifestyle and labor market composition. Though coming chapters will consider the popular condemnations of the overweight body as undisciplined and unproductive, for now, note the paradox: though food writers and cultural critics trace rising obesity rates to changing economic factors (sedentary lifestyles, working mothers, fast food, etc.), the privatization of food informs a widespread assumption that the *cure* for obesity lies in a return to individual responsibility. This prescription seems but one manifestation of a common trend: the privatization of concerns raised by massive economic transformations.

Taking a longer look at food history, however, we can see that the privatization of food far precedes the cultural politics of the postwar United States. Though critiques of this privatization invariably focus on the past few decades, the argument could easily be pushed back another fifty years, as Richard Bulliet shows in his focus on the urbanization process that removed agricultural concerns from the daily lives of most Americans.[29] Living in cities instead of on farms, consumers came to see eating as the intake of so much standardized and impersonal fuel, an economic transaction, instead of one moment in an ethical bond between humans, animals, and land; eating appears as a part of household or bodily management, more like bathing or vacuuming than communing with nature. For Bulliet, food was not privatized in the postwar period when families stopped eating together, but in what he calls the "post-domestic" period in which people no longer had any immediate relationship to the production of their own food.

Each of these arguments is essentially technological, focusing on how changes in the production, processing, and distribution of food made it practical for people to eat alone. Certainly, the widespread availability of packaged, standardized, and relatively nonperishable food items marks a significant break from a world in which people participate in the industrial, organic, and laboring practices that convert seed, soil, water, and sunlight into edible proteins. And just as certainly, the pace of (post) industrial life all but demands a reliance on packaged, processed, or fast food. But what is missing in these arguments is a consideration of why the possibility of a private cuisine would be desirable—why the celebration of pleasure of public eating would succumb to the convenience and pragmatism of eating alone.

In the first half of this book, I aim to demonstrate that the privatization of food was an essential moment in the rise of modern liberalism. The discourse of the sovereign self animating seventeenth-century political theory had profound implications on social understandings of food, as the practice of eating was transformed from a traditionally public engagement into a quintessentially private activity. Alongside the enclosures of public land, the expansion of capitalist markets, and principled extension of religious tolerance, the architects of modern liberalism (René Descartes, Thomas Hobbes, and John Locke) were preoccupied with defining and maintaining a border between the self and the world, informally relegating substances that confound that border (most notably, food) to an increasingly crucial private sphere. In other words, as liberal politics pursued an expansion of the private sphere at the expense of the public, the metabolic demands of the body found themselves absorbed into this expanded private sphere. This, I claim, was no mere coincidence. This shunting of food from the public sphere resonated with an emergent idea of individual selves that was necessary to legitimate a mode of governance organized under the banner of a social contract. That is, the social contract—as a political metaphor—requires particular types of subjects that I aim to show were uncomfortable with and increasingly disgusted by the material transactions characteristic of the process of digestion.

I argue that the privatization of food that is typically located in the past half century is just the latest stage in a long process of removing from public life the concerns and realities of the lived body. I further argue that food discourse today is similarly occupied with contesting or reifying the border that separates the self from the other. Just as social order of the seventeenth century came increasingly to depend on the clean division of spaces—from territories and houses to laboratories and bathrooms—the world of the twenty-first century is seeing radical challenges to that order. Anxieties about national sovereignty, international immigration, and personal privacy all trade in a concern about the ability to maintain these borders. The discourses of food on display today reflect anxieties about the collapse of these and other precious borders: borders between the self and the other, borders between states, and borders between the human and the nonhuman—or as I will put it, the borders of self, space, and species.

Given the degree to which political thought and social life of the past four centuries has relied on the existence of clear borders—borders between the self and the world, borders between public and private spaces, borders between sovereign states, and borders between human and nonhuman—it is not mere hyperbole to claim, as many critics do, that the challenges to those borders comprising globalization constitute a threat to our very ability to conceptualize political order.[30] If established vocabularies of objectivity, property, and sovereignty depend on these borders, what do we do without them? I argue that food anxieties reflect this collapse of meaning, this challenge to our political vocabulary. Further, in absence of these reliable borders, we have floundered through attempts to develop a political vocabulary adequate to the task of democracy.

As a result, so much discourse about food and politics surrounds attempts to shore up these borders. At the global level, the international Slow Food movement emphasizes the importance of *terroir*, the material linkage to a territorial space, just as nativist identity movements, border vigilantism, and regional agreements like NAFTA and the EU all seek to reinforce the traditional significance of lived space and the borders between spaces. At the individual level, the U.S. government passed the Personal Responsibility in Food Consumption Act (a.k.a. "The Cheeseburger Bill") in 2003, reinforcing the American ideology of individual responsibility by officially refusing to hold producers or vendors of fattening foods liable for causing obesity, while the food activism largely associated with the work of Michael Pollan promises a return to a Jeffersonian ideal of self-reliant individuals through backyard gardening, home cooking, and responsible consumerism. In each case, an earlier border, now threatened by the forces of globalization and corporate capitalism, is retrieved and reinforced.

While the reinforcement of national borders with walls, police, and armed vigilantes is the most obvious manifestation of this anxiety, the consumerist tone of so much food activism reveals just how thoroughly privatized politics can become, with public health and global inequality supposedly remediated by a diligent pursuit of individual integrity. That liberal societies have experienced a progressive decline in public life as more issues became private is, of course, an old claim.[31] The idea that citizens of liberal societies have come to see political activity through the lens of the market, with the rise of the "citizen consumer" through the twentieth century, is slightly more recent but also hardly new.[32] But the current popularity of "green" or "responsible" consumerism—in which such pressing issues as climate change and the decline in national sovereignty can be addressed through wise consumer choices (*vote with your dollar!*)—is notable for the hegemony that the idea maintains over the political discourse today. Pollan, for instance, characterizes buying foods from a local provider rather than Wal-Mart as "a kind of civic act, even a form of protest," and even goes so far as to call it "a linchpin of [the] rebellion" against an exploitative industrial economy.[33] In so conflating political rebellion and informed shopping, Pollan provides confirmation of Wendy Brown's thesis that neoliberalism extends market rationality to all domains of social and political life, undermining the "relative autonomy of certain institutions from one another and from the market . . . that formerly sustained an interval and a tension between capitalist political economy and a liberal democratic political system."[34]

Leaving aside for now the presumed *efficacy* of consumerist politics, consider its appeal. In an era with limited trust in public institutions and in which citizen activity is filtered through understandings of the market, Pollan becomes an international political celebrity by directing attention to the one realm where citizens can still imagine exercising power: the market. Just as the official politics of obesity reinforces a discourse of individual responsibility right when people feel so powerless in the face of economic power, consumerist politics valorize committed action in the private sphere when the institutions of public power seem unresponsive to popular appeals. Just as food itself was privatized, today even food *politics* is privatized, an activity to be indulged at home, or between the consumer and the producer, with little or no intervention of public institutions. In this advanced stage of neoliberalism, Berry's linking food choice to agricultural production is subject to a curious inversion: not only does eating have political effects, but eating is also characterized as an engagement in politics itself. Grocery shopping, or caring for the household, gets elevated to the status of political action. Berry's politicization of consumption, in other words, is transformed into a consumerizationof politics.

States of Sovereignty

In coming chapters, I will be arguing that the politicization of consumer activity is a logical response to a real erosion of the traditional sites and mechanisms of political power under neoliberalism. Most broadly, I will argue that the concentrations of power and the distributions of resources have contributed to both a sense and an actuality of powerlessness—a loss of national sovereignty as states grow beholden to the dictates of global corporations and international finance organizations, and a simultaneous loss of individual sovereignty as more and more of our lives are controlled by distant and anonymous institutions. With little or no faith in states to represent our interests, and with economic and political power eclipsed by that of large organizations, citizens have turned their attention to the one domain in which they can still imagine wielding power: the market. More than a distraction from the real sites of politics, I argue, this consumerist turn is part of the political apparatus of neoliberalism, affording subjects the power and the desire to govern themselves (and each other) through informal mechanisms of ethical regard and voluntary contract in a manner that confers legitimacy on a political arrangement that proves increasingly incapable of satisfying the needs and desires of vast numbers of people.

Certainly, this is not always the case. Some contributions to food politics—most notably those deploying terms like *food sovereignty* and *food democracy*—freely invoke the urgency of political reforms regarding systems of land allocation and intellectual property for addressing ongoing injustices and predicted food crises.[35] But more frequently, the voices and texts of food politics rely on an apolitical language of individual choice to propose solutions to some of the more entrenched dilemmas facing a global society. Generally, this default to a consumerist politics seems to stem from either a desire to be pragmatic or a failure of political imagination. But another reason for this restriction of political discourse can be inferred from the frequency with which diet manuals and food treatises appeal to a wounded notion of trust. Michael Pollan's indictment of "Big Organic" in *The Omnivore's Dilemma* and his subsequent celebration of traditional diets in *Food Rules* both turn on a claim that we cannot trust the federal government, nutrition scientists, or the food industry to help us find nourishing and responsible food.[36] Marion Nestle argues that "Big Food" has completely corrupted federal dietary guidelines, while obesity skeptics trace our dietary commonsense to a fashion industry, a "dietary pharmaceutical complex," or a "health industrial complex" that have been proven more adept at and interested in producing profits than health.[37] Barry Glassner summarily argues that dietary science, federal guidelines, and marketing appeals are all ultimately unreliable, and so we might as well just eat whatever makes us happy.[38] Perhaps most explicitly, *New York Times* science writer and America's leading carb vilifier Gary Taubes indicts medical professionals, nutrition scientists, and the U.S. Department of Agriculture for actually recommending the very diets that cause not only obesity but also a wealth of "diseases of civilization" from diabetes and hypertension to ulcers and varicose veins.[39]

Such widespread skepticism signals not just a crisis of diet and nutritional information but a crisis of confidence in the institutions traditionally charged with ensuring public safety—especially government and the institutions of medical and dietary science. Hence the pronounced libertarian streak in so much food writing, with exhortations to bypass federal regulators and buy food that is "beyond organic," to decide for yourself what is a healthy weight, or to look to tradition or grandparents rather than the government for guidance on what to eat. Such privatized decision making more or less explicitly declares that, given the track record of these institutions, you can only take care of yourself. In which case, this is not a crisis surrounding food; rather, the discourse of food is one symptom of a political crisis surrounding issues of legitimacy, trust, representation, and (most broadly) sovereignty.

The paradox, however, is that just as the literature calls into question the reliability of formal institutions, it simultaneously relies on and calls into question the narrative of the sovereign individual. The metaphorics of digestion, as we will soon see, has long served to question this grounding myth of political liberalism. In coming chapters, I will argue that just as White and Connolly suggest that recognizing one's essential vulnerability informs a different, more generous approach to politics, food literature often appeals precisely because it draws attention to a particular moment when the ideal of sovereign individuality breaks down. In eating, that is, we are revealed as vulnerable, needy, dependent creatures rather than the rational and autonomous selves of liberal discourse. I will

argue that food literature of recent years—and here I mean both the popularity of food writers like Michael Pollan and also the increased attention
to food in academic discourses across the liberal arts and humanities—
concentrates a general anxiety about this ideal and therefore the political
ideal of national sovereignty and representative government it supports.
Food literature calls attention to the tenuousness of the very terms we
have for understanding power, politics, and democracy. In other words, I
will argue that food occupies a central position in our political discourse
because it is the site at which our corporeal integrity is most visibly called
into question and, as such, the site at which the anxieties surrounding
this integrity and its attainability coalesce. It is no mere coincidence, I
argue, that these concerns have grown so prominent in this current neoliberal moment.

Both of these crises—the crisis of individual sovereignty and the crisis
of national sovereignty—are on display in the heated debates over obesity rates in the United States. At the individual level, arguments about
the causes and the treatments for obesity clearly center on the question
of the degree to which individuals can and should be held responsible
for their own dietary and health care choices. While nutritionists like
Kelly Brownell and Marion Nestle point to a "toxic food environment"
in which the national government and medical professionals, co-opted
by corporate lobbying and sponsorship, no longer represent the needs
of the citizens but rather of corporations,[40] the moral judgment laid on
the overweight turns entirely on their presumed lack of self-control. This
ideological bifurcation was only intensified in 2003, when the U.S. government passed the Cheeseburger Bill, which either (depending on one's
perspective) bolstered the nation's commitment to personal responsibility or manifest the blatant corruption of Congress by moneyed interests.
But this is significantly complicated by the recent classification of obesity as an "epidemic," which is subject to medical and epidemiological
treatment. Add to this the realization that the highest concentrations of
obesity in the United States are among nonwhite and immigrant populations (often along the U.S.–Mexico border), and the obesity debates are
suddenly implicated in discourses of race, immigration, border security,
and national identity.

In short, what is at stake in the debates about obesity is not just public
health and fitness but the enduring viability of such seemingly indispensable concepts as agency, responsibility, and sovereignty. Each of these
concepts has similarly been subject to renewed attention from social

theorists seeking to salvage them from the dustbin of history as the onto-logical assumptions underwriting them come under heavy fire.[41] I argue that food literature carries such currency today because it speaks directly to concerns about sovereignty and powerlessness by promising a mea-sure of personal and local control via individual choice and responsible consumerism. But this is a limited and often incoherent idea of control, appealing as it often does to precisely the language of sovereignty that is itself in question. Thus the underlying project of *Eating Anxiety* is to examine the material threats to the ideals of sovereignty that seem so indispensable to political order, to examine the anxieties provoked by these threats, and, ultimately, to explore the political efficacy of what I call the digestive subjectivity that emerges from the discourse of food.

The Question of Method

Reading the long history of scholarship about food, one notes trends and genres that both exemplify and codify vocabularies for thinking about politics. One popular genre chooses a particular food (sugar, corn, or salt, for example) and explores how that food changed history.[42] Another genre inverts this strategy, explaining how massive historical develop-ments (the invention of the automobile, democracy, or plastic) changed the way we eat.[43] A third, more recent genre turns from history to politi-cal economy, exploring commodity chains in which a particular finished product (coffee or sushi) is revealed for its implication in exploitative or destructive practices in distant locals.[44] Reading this literature, some interesting methodological issues arise. Compare, for instance, two dif-ferent approaches from notable food historians to the same priggish question: Why is the American cuisine so bland? Margaret Visser chalks this up to an American egalitarianism (spicy or exotic foods are too exclu-sionary) and argues that an emergent popularity of "nouvelle cuisine" owes to the breakdown of cultural hegemony signaled by the term "post-modernism."[45] By contrast, Harvey Levenstein traces this blandness to the explosion in packaged foods through the twentieth century, such that food companies had to produce bland foods if they were to appeal to as wide a market as possible.[46] Such different theses rely on very specific and very significant ideas about history and culture, as well as the rela-tive power of ideal and material forces. But the ultimate payoff of these studies—those explaining how food changed history, those explaining how history changed food, and those explaining how food arrived at your plate—are roughly the same: a cultural explanation for why we eat a certain way.

My aim is somewhat different. The payoff of *Eating Anxiety* is less historical than philosophical and less cultural than political. My wager is that particular ways of thinking about the activity of eating provoke different ways of thinking about knowledge, identity, and power. In this sense, books about food offer fertile ground for thinking about the operations and significance of epistemology, ethics, and politics. Necessarily drawing on and reinforcing as they do specific ideas about bodies and force, they allow or disallow particular ways of thinking about freedom, coercion, and opportunity. My aim in this book, therefore, is not to explain how or why we eat as we do, but rather to explain how representations of what it means to be a being that eats have profound implications on how we understand such perennial issues as property ownership, individual responsibility, and the possibility and desirability of democratic rule.

One route to making this argument is through attention to political metaphors. For instance, when Hobbes (despite his manifest critique of the use of metaphor in politics) describes the Leviathan as an "Artificiall Man," when Marx describes commerce as "social metabolism," and when the U.S. surgeon general describes obesity as an "epidemic," each draws on and conveys a particular understanding of bodies, force, and causality. Similarly, the terms "body politic" and "social contract" both convey nontrivial assumptions about the constitution of society, with the organic and essential connotations of the former standing in stark contrast with the legalistic and voluntaristic connotations of the latter. These metaphors—as well as their more contemporary rival, "social network"— function as what Lakoff and Johnson call "structural metaphors," which use one highly delineated concept to organize our understanding of another, such that society itself appears in one instance as a living organism, in another as a legal arrangement, and in the third as a loose and ever-evolving web.[47]

With this consideration of metaphor in mind, *Eating Anxiety* does not pursue a cultural explanation of why we eat a certain way, but rather argues that cultural narratives of food and eating provide us with some of our most deeply held convictions about what it means to be a political agent. In this, narratives of food and eating are decidedly material, in that they orient us to the world and produce particular kinds of subjects (entitled or ascetic, imperious or vulnerable, joyful or anxious). The underlying stakes, then, surround the relation of political language (and political theory) to political practice. Not reducible to either an "idealist" or a "materialist" account in which language either constructs or reflects reality, I argue that the canonical figures in political theory (e.g., Hobbes, Locke, Marx, and Nietzsche) provide vocabularies for thinking about selves, spaces, and species that have crucial impacts on how people come to experience and understand politics. Further, much of the political hand-wringing going on today (from academic debates about agency and sovereignty to popular debates about responsibility and immigration) owe in large part to the fact that contemporary developments in philosophy, science, commerce, and technology threaten to undermine the vocabularies used to conceptualize politics. In other words, what I am calling the anxieties of globalization arise from a sense that the established vocabularies of politics seem no longer adequate to explain or organize the contemporary world, and what I am calling digestive subjectivity offers an increasingly compelling response to this inadequacy.

To be clear, I am not reading these texts—whether Hobbes's *Leviathan*, Nietzsche's *Genealogy of Morals*, or Pollan's *The Omnivore's Dilemma*—as authoritative documents of their respective eras. Rather, I am reading them as inroads to understanding traditions of thought, and suggesting that canonical texts, as evidenced by their becoming canonical, provide ways of thinking about problems and relations that are satisfying to large numbers of people. They establish or reinforce particular ways of understanding the world—which, as I will discuss more in Chapter 1, is what I take Marx to be describing with the term "ideology." I therefore read these texts and their metaphors for what they provide *implicitly*. So while the primary task of Locke's *Second Treatise* is not to convince the reader of an ontology, I argue that the persuasive force of that text comes from its providing (or corresponding to) a way of understanding the nature of being and, more specifically, a way of understanding identity, space, and species. Further, I argue that what makes Locke one of the architects of contemporary political ideology is less his theory of property than his underlying and implicit explanation of what it means to be a political agent. My point in reading Locke, in other words, is not to suss out the value of his theory of property but to show how his theory of property is predicated on a theory of subjectivity that continues to structure how we encounter the material world.

Similarly, Nietzsche, in the passages previously quoted, uses food not exactly as a metaphor but as a metonym for the processes of life itself. Digesting, learning, acculturating—these are all processes of consuming and appropriating the outside world, blurring the boundary between outside and inside. His work shows how eating—like any experiential activity that leaves a mark on the subject—is necessarily thick with concerns about individual sovereignty, the manipulation of nature, and the ethics of killing other things. The flip side, of course, is to realize that our bodies and minds are assaulted on a persistent basis by other forces—from microbes to amino acids to marketing messages to loved ones—seeking their own survival, causing the suffering that Nietzsche diagnoses is the sine qua non of life itself. These paired messages (i.e., that humans are essentially power hungry and that personal identity is a function of violation) are what have allowed so many and incompatible appropriations of Nietzsche, as the patron saint of both fascism and radical democracy.

For reasons stated earlier, I focus specifically on discourses and metaphors of food because they prove useful for unpacking the operations of ideology. That is, because eating constitutes such an intimate engagement with other beings and the material world, the discourse of eating consolidates and intensifies broader feelings about the relations between self and other, between public and private, and between human and nonhuman. As Kass puts this, "eating as such reveals the paradoxical and problematic relationship between any living being and the rest of the world; for in eating, each living being homogenizes other forms and denies other life, appropriating them solely for its own use and purpose."[48] Following Nietzsche, we might respond that this is the case for any act of consumption from shopping to reading. But unlike buying a Prius or a plot of land, in which the object of consumption becomes appended to or a prosthetic of the body, when we eat, the object of consumption is actually incorporated into the self. As Kass notes, eating thus not only helps constitute the self but also constitutes one's *sense of* self, provoking reflection on who we are, how we act, what it means to be an individual, what it means to be a person, and what it means to be free. For this reason, I argue, the debates about species purity on display in debates about genetically modified organisms, for instance, are but intensified versions of anxieties found across society—in debates about Darwin, for instance. Methodologically, my claim reflects that of Mary Douglas, who reads concerns about dirt as symptoms of broader concerns about social disorder and the borders of the body as metonymical for other borders and protocols that govern social relations.[49] Here, I argue that anxieties about food reflect broader anxieties about the categories used to maintain political order: specifically, anxieties about the enduring reliability of the liberal ideals of individual and national sovereignty.

Much of my point can be stated as follows: many contemporary food discourses—from nutritional attention to the role of hormones in regulating weight to the valorization of farmers' markets as sites of community to concerns about the ethics of killing animals for food—are rooted in anxieties about a series of challenges to liberal politics by technological, economic, and cultural forces of globalization. In other words, as the forces of globalization disrupt the established institutions charged with organizing political life, subjects experience anxiety as the concepts traditionally charged with organizing political life (responsibility, representation, and sovereignty) become less adequate to the task. As citizens and philosophers wrestle with the pressing question of how our organizing political metaphor—now a "social network" rather than a "social contract"—might inform political life, discourses of food both redirect that anxiety and also help establish another mode of social organization, all under the manageable and neoliberal vocabulary of individual choice.

This book thus reckons not only with different texts but also with different kinds of texts, from historical political treatises to contemporary popular polemics. Sometimes this reckoning happens within a single chapter, but more often, it happens across chapters. In each case, the aim is to show how these texts provide us with terms and frameworks that will organize our thoughts and institutions. These frameworks can be seen animating broad cultural trends across different fields, from science and politics to ethics and aesthetics. The aim in exploring writers like Michael Pollan in light of writers like Nietzsche, in other words, is not to issue the summary reading of either but to show how both help to produce the ontopolitical vocabularies that we use to organize our experience.

Bill of Fare

Because this book is a work of political theory, attempting to show how developments in political thought help explain broader cultural movements and artifacts, the book itself alternates between textual explication and cultural criticism. Some might find this organization (rather than a strictly chronological argument) disorienting. But my hope is that by organizing the text this way, readers will be convinced of the relevance of the more historical examination of political treatises to the more topical analysis of contemporary food debates. The payoff, I hope, is that even if Locke or Hobbes make scant appearance in the chapter on obesity (for instance), my earlier readings of how they figured the human body can be seen to influence how we experience and respond to such public health issues. The final chapter of the book reconciles these two approaches, showing how the material covered in the first six chapters contributes to the field of democratic theory.

Chapter 1 uses the discourse of diet to organize an understanding of the relationship between the scientific understanding of bodies and political ideology. Chronicling three periods of dietary advice in the United States over the twentieth century and indexing these periods to distinct paradigms of production and capitalist accumulation, I show how programs like Weight Watchers and the Atkins diet captured particular anxieties about freedom and self-reliance, while also contributing to a technique of population management that Foucault calls biopolitics.

Chapter 2, "Eating Alone" moves back to the seventeenth century to explore the rise of the liberal subjectivity that is presumed in the dietary advice discussed in chapter 1. This chapter explores canonical texts of liberal thought as well as popular contributions to food ethics to show how a particular model of the sovereign individual was constructed by masking digestive processes. Chapter 3 examines a subsequent *un*masking of these processes in scientific, aesthetic, and political discourse of the nineteenth century. Identifying what I call the "digestive turn" in political thought, I show how G. W. F. Hegel, Karl Marx, and Friedrich Nietzsche used digestive metaphors to disrupt the ontopolitical assumptions of liberalism, thus disrupting the ideals of value, subjectivity, and work that underwrite the social contract.

Chapters 4 and 5 turn to contemporary food politics to explore how debates about obesity and local foods at the opening of the twenty-first century betray twin crises in the traditional ideals of individual and national sovereignty. Here I trace both crises to technological and political challenges to the partition of space on which liberal order depends, and I show how classifications of obesity and the valorization of local foods both attempt to reinforce threatened borders that have been used to legitimate democratic governance. Chapter 6 turns to the discourse of species, and explores how anxieties about the production and consumption of meat reflect the technological and philosophical challenges to humanism that similarly underwrite liberal politics. Together, these chapters reveal anxieties about three cherished categories—self, space, and species—that are presumed by dominant narratives about representative politics, capitalist markets, and individual responsibility.

The conclusion, "Democracy and Disgust," ties together the theoretical and the topical chapters by using the sentiment of disgust to explore the engagement of the other that is required in democratic practice. Having traced a certain fear of the body to a sterile ideal of a transcendent subject in chapter 2, this chapter mobilizes the insights of subsequent chapters to explore the idea of a "digestive subject," which is more attuned to the vulnerability and corporeality of human life. I argue that this model of subjectivity offers some resources for creating a more robust commitment to collective living but lacks the necessary political purchase to anchor a properly democratic theory.

A Word on Scope

At first glance, this book might seem overly broad and unfocused, covering issues as disparate as the metaphors of digestion in the history of political thought to an evolutionary aversion to feces to the ethics of animal cloning. From another perspective, however, the study might seem restrictively narrow. This book is firmly rooted in a tradition of politics that I hope will be familiar to most readers but which is, admittedly, quite recent on the political landscape. It touches only incidentally on the role of food in religious practices (and when it does, it is restricted almost exclusively to Christianity). It also largely ignores numerous pressing food issues such as peasant land reform politics and the enduring threats of famine.

If one were to embark on a comprehensive study of food politics, however, one would quickly be overwhelmed by the sheer volume of texts and issues. As such, this study is quite specifically focused on the role of food in what readers will recognize as a modern, liberal worldview. Elsewhere, I have described that worldview as postmetaphysical commitment to identity (consistency of personhood), authenticity (internal sovereignty of the self over the I), and responsibility (a meritorious allocation of punishments and rewards).[50] This study continues with that description, and my argument turns on the belief that the institutions and practices of everyday life in the United States at the opening of the twenty-first century are largely anchored in this worldview.

It may also be said that my analysis, at times, lacks sufficient attention to subjective dimensions of class, race, gender, and sexuality. By talking about what food (or obesity, or cannibalism, or community) means to people, I might be passing over the very real and unavoidable fact it surely means different things to different people, and that these differences are not random but quite systematic. But often the subjects and movements being described in this book are idealized versions of same, and it is by now well rehearsed that such ideals themselves are presumed to lack a class, a race, a gender, or a sexuality. Indeed, insofar as what is being described (particularly in the first two chapters) is the emergence of a liberal subject that is ashamed of its own hunger, the aggressive masking of characteristics of the body is not only incidental but also fundamental to the operations involved. That is, not only should it be familiar by now that the liberal subject presumes itself abstract and universal, I am arguing that that abstraction and universality actually depends on a more or less sustained neglect of the mechanics (and specific markings) of bodies. The aim of the current project, in other words, is to examine both the origins and the operations of this abstraction, to highlight its mechanics and its markings, and to see what it can and what it cannot do. Only then, perhaps, will we see what is required to develop a taste for democracy.

1   DIET AND AMERICAN IDEOLOGY

PERHAPS THE BEST PLACE TO start a study of eating and sovereignty is with the discourse of diet, where food and control converge in an ideological matrix of individual responsibility, self-mastery, and population management. Studies of famines or agricultural labor can reveal some of the ways that the production, distribution, and regulation of food manifest political power at the level of the individual body. But dietary advice and particular weight loss regimens can most clearly demonstrate how the demands of political order are personalized in liberal society. In this chapter, I show how diet trends of the past century have participated in dominant political economic trends and have helped to fashion the kinds of entrepreneurial subjects required for the advancement of neoliberal capitalism.[1]

Dieting, it has been noted, is as American as apple pie. And though cynics tend to read the ever-proliferating number of diet fads as a series of pseudoscientific schemes marketed to the gullible, the ideal of dieting seems but one instance of a narrative of self-mastery that is the hallmark of American political ideology. Various studies have questioned dietary literature for providing an ideal of individual self-control, precisely as a retreat from domains of politics and economics in which people feel powerless. But this chapter seeks to go further, explaining dietary literature not as a *displacement* or an *escape* from politics, but as a shifted terrain of politics itself. As a brand of self-help literature that embodies a subtle and sophisticated technique of population management, dietary literature actually intensifies—rather than distracts from—politics.

This chapter also demonstrates the methodological approach of this book as a whole, reading both canonical and academic texts alongside popular narratives of the individual body in order to demonstrate how the mechanisms of political power manifest in commonsense under-standings and individual habits. Looking at one very specific piece of this story—diet trends through the twentieth-century United States—this chapter argues that often unstated ideas about the individual body cor-respond to broader and more abstract notions about politics, freedom, and the relative power of ideals, will, and matter. The point of bringing these disparate archives into contact is to show how discourses of food constitute particular types of subjects with particular desires, abilities, and expectations.

This chapter thus takes an unconventional approach to a very con-ventional question: *What diets work?* Examined politically, a diet can be said to work *not* when it helps somebody achieve a desired biolog-ical goal, but when it provides a satisfying way of understanding the human body.[2] That is, diets *work* when they achieve a kind of popularity approaching commonsense—as what happened when Americans gen-erally accepted the idea that counting calories, suppressing appetite, or avoiding carbohydrates would allow them to lose weight. The chap-ter thus explores diets as ideology, as frameworks for understanding the operation of their own bodies, and the functioning of systems of value and mobility more generally. This chapter explores this question—*What diets work?*—with specific attention on three popular approaches to diet over the past century, from the earliest advice about regulating caloric energy to the commercially successful endeavors of Weight Watchers and the Atkins diet. These specific examples are illustrative not only because they prove to be the most "successful" diet discourses of the past century but because they also stand in for larger trends in dietary common-sense that can be indexed to broader cultural and political phenomena. In particular, in these three types of advice, one can see personalized and directed narratives about the political and economic requirements of specific stages in the development of the American economy, from a vibrant driver of an industrial development to a reluctant participant in a global information economy.

The Structure of Dietetic Revolutions

In *The Structure of Scientific Revolutions*, Thomas Kuhn debunks the notion of the history of science as a linear, progressive movement toward truth, identifying instead a series of momentous "paradigm shifts" in which radically new understandings of the world compete with more familiar metascientific assumptions for cultural and institutional hegemony.[3] The most familiar of these battles is when Copernicus, in the face of scientific and religious orthodoxy, proposed a heliocentric view of the universe—a view that found increasing acceptance in the scientific community as more and more empirical evidence was found to support it over the prevailing geocentrism. Kuhn himself admits that he uses the example of the Copernican Revolution reluctantly; it is too obvious to avoid, but astronomy, a discipline necessarily invested in passive and prosaic notions of observation, is less than ideal for demonstrating his broader thesis: that scientific discoveries do not merely entail refinement and improvement over old ways of knowing such that the scientific community is progressively moving toward truth, but rather that "paradigms" carry unstated and extrascientific assumptions that color what investigators will see through scientific investigation. As such, Kuhn argues that all paradigms offer intriguing but incomplete knowledge of the phenomena they seek to explain. For this reason, paradigms compete for hegemony in the scientific community, and new paradigms replace older ones when they are shown to afford more satisfying resources for framing scientific questions.

Kuhn's thesis seems tailor-made to understanding fits and starts of American dietary advice. While most new diet plans constitute minor and aesthetic variations on familiar themes (*eat fewer calories* or *raise your metabolism*, etc.), we can identify a number of developments that we can, following Kuhn and without bombast, call "dietetic revolutions," in which the fundamental assumptions underlying established ideas about weight management were challenged by novel paradigms that eventually established cultural hegemony. John Coveney, relying primarily on volumes two and three of Foucault's *History of Sexuality*, chronicles a shift between ancient Greek and Roman worldviews (where discourse of food was thick with moral considerations about self-restraint and fitness for rule) and modern Christian and Enlightenment worldviews (where diet and weight became primarily subjects of scientific knowledge).[4] Similarly, Anson Rabinbach discusses how the discovery of thermodynamics in the nineteenth century fundamentally changed approaches to food; hereafter, physicists came to understand the body as a "human motor" that could be regulated (and exhausted) just as mechanical machinery could.[5] Rabinbach's thesis will return at length in chapter 3. For now, it will suffice to note that just as Copernicus did not merely move the earth, but rather offered "a whole new way of regarding the problem of physics and astronomy, one that necessarily changed the meaning of both 'earth' and 'motion,'"[6] these developments—from a spiritual to a moral and then to a mechanical explanation of diet—did not merely change our diet but offered whole new ways of regarding bodies and desire. They, in turn, provoked allied shifts in discourses of ethics, politics, and aesthetics.

In Kuhn's argument, new paradigms replace older paradigms when they are shown to have greater explanatory power. But conversation across paradigms is often crippled by a lack of shared assumptions—for instance, those who see depression as a function of a chemical imbalance have little to say to those committed to more sociological explanations, and neither can communicate clearly with those who see depression as punishment for sin. As Kuhn puts it, "the proponents of competing paradigms practice their trades in different worlds. . . . Practicing in different worlds, the two groups of scientists see different things when they look for the same point in the same direction."[7]

In terms of diet, the disconnect often surrounds not merely what is a healthy body weight but, as the familiar dietary refrain of "mind over matter" suggests, broader existential disagreements about the nature of the individual, the possibility of free will, and the relative importance of ideas, materiality, and desire for determining the course of life. Whether someone sees body weight as a function of virtue, metabolism, or genetics, for instance, says less about the actual processes of weight gain than it does about their assumptions regarding causality, value, and blame. While Kuhn explains the difficulty in collaborating across these assumptions, what he does not explore is *why* some assumptions might rise to cultural hegemony—what material or sociological factors might, for instance, render a population ready to believe one set of assumption at the cost of other.[8]

Following Max Weber, we might explore how successful discourses of diet have an "elective affinity" with other narratives of success that help organize society.[9] Dietary ideas about will power, for instance, might resonate with spiritual discourses about self-restraint or economic discourses about frugality that are endemic to both the Protestant ethic and the spirit of capitalism. In a Weberian vein, diets are successful not when they prove themselves empirically effective but when their animating concepts and metaphors are consistent with and amplify broader assumptions about meaning and success. Since the mid-nineteenth century, popular approaches to diet have been organized primarily not around moral issues like gluttony or sin but rather hegemonic economic ideas—especially economic calculations of a body's energy needs and uses.[10] As nutritionist Marion Nestle often puts it in simple and familiar terms, "[t]he cause of overweight" is not laziness, gluttony, or fate, but rather and simply "an excess of calories consumed over calories burned off in activity."[11] Twentieth-century diet literature, that is, operates with a thoroughly rationalized body that can be controlled, predicted, and manipulated with the established techniques of medical and economic science.

For Foucault, this capture of diet by an economic and medical science corresponds to the rise not only of the human sciences and industrialization but to a mode of control in which people are given the tools and the motivations to govern themselves. It corresponds to the rise of a series of techniques and discourses that have been enacted at the level of the individual body and also at the social body to effect a manageable, predictable, and productive population—to manage "the controlled insertion of bodies into the machinery of production and the adjustment of the phenomena of population to economic processes."[12] Biopower, Foucault writes, "brought life and its mechanisms into the realm of explicit calculations and made knowledge-power an agent of transformation of human life."[13] From this perspective, the capture of diet by economics is less interesting than the proliferation of dietary discourse in general, such that managing one's weight became a tool of self-governance, and individuals were afforded both the ability and the motivation to ensure the productive and predictable development of their own body toward the end of smooth economic development. For Foucault, the proliferation of dietary discourse is part and parcel of the rise of modern liberalism, where the knowledge of the human sciences coincided with the privatization of economic and political power, such that the tools and practices of dietary regulation help to produce the very kind of self-reliant and entrepreneurial subjects needed by a capitalist economy.[14]

Chronicling a year in a commercial weight loss program, Cressida Heyes details just this kind of self-surveillance and self-discipline that entrepreneurial capitalism requires.[15] Unlike the closely monitored and hierarchically supervised subjects of Foucault's *Discipline and Punish*, Heyes describes dieters monitoring themselves—keeping detailed records of meals, activities, moods, and weights—all toward the end of better self-awareness and, thus, self-control. (In some organizations, like Weight Watchers, dieters even offer weekly confessional progress reports.) As Barbara Cruikshank puts this in an analysis of an allied "self esteem" movement, these discourses of self-improvement are "practical technolog[ies] for the production of certain kinds of selves"—in particular, selves that "recognize, isolate, and act upon their own subjectivity" so that they can be "governors of their own selves."[16] Dieting, particularly as it is concentrated among women, drags a vital population into the domain of biopolitics—a population less subject to the disciplinary force of so many other institutions like factories and prisons. In the popular weight loss regimes as promoted by organizations such as Weight Watchers and Jenny Craig, the individual body and soul, through a narrative of self-discovery and self-control, becomes the territory on which politics takes place.[17] Creating subjects that can be held responsible for their choices and their health, such organizations promise not so much slenderness as self-mastery. As I will discuss in coming chapters, the overweight (read: unmanaged) body is increasingly subject to political scrutiny through the twentieth century for its failure to become the sovereign individual on which a liberal economy depends.[18]

The capture of diet by the discourse of economics, thus, corresponds to a privatization of political power under the guise of liberalism. From within this economic discourse, diet is the management of energy transactions between the self and the world—in other words, another form of labor.[19] Whereas in conventional labor this transaction happens as the self extends itself into the world, diet moves the space of labor to the internal domain of the individual body; it is intensive (rather than extensive) labor. Susan Bordo has long talked about diet in this way: not the regulated expression of the self into the world, but the regulated expression of the world into the self.[20] Seeing diet as just another form of domestic work, it makes sense that the discourse of diet has been largely associated with women, who have long been largely excluded from the realms of extensive labor (economics and politics). Indeed, psychologists, psychiatrists, nutritionists, and philosophers have been arguing for decades that the most extreme and pathological forms of diet (eating disorders such as anorexia nervosa) are less about food than about control, and that the concentration of eating disorders among women owes to the fact that men have been afforded greater opportunities to express a desire for control via productive labor in traditional labor markets and the domination of women.[21] Bordo even suggests that the eating disorders afflicting so many young women in the 1970s might owe to the frustrated experiences of women's liberation, with the sixties promises of equality and fulfillment for women butting up against an impacted labor market unable to provide it.[22]

In this light, the heightened attention to men's bodies and the defeminization of diet in recent years, which Bordo examines in *The Male Body*, can be seen as a symptom of a declining sense of economic agency among men. Probably the best marker of the defeminization of diet is the rise of lite beer and diet soda in the 1970s. Though lite beer was unheard of in the early 1970s, by the end of the decade no televised sporting event was complete without a few memorable reminders that even the burliest of men can watch their figure while drinking beer. Similarly, though the Coca-Cola Company had been selling diet soda under the name TaB since 1963, it was not until 1982 that the company felt safe to tarnish its brand with something called "Diet Coke."[23] As postwar prosperity began to fade, with family wages and job security in steady decline, the discourse of diet steadily expanded to offer men (as well as women) the opportunity for self-mastery. An increased fascination with male bodies and diets, evident in an intensified commitment to exercise and the idealized representations of the male body in popular culture, in other words, offer solace from the loss of economic and political power that define so much of the terrain of American masculinity.[24] Ironically, however, they reinforce discourses of self-sufficiency that continue to legitimate a cutthroat economic environment.

Paradigms of the Twentieth Century

Hillel Schwartz's *Never Satisfied* is widely credited as a (if not the) canonical text in critical diet literature. That book presents the diet industry as moving from one dubious scheme to another in perpetual pursuit of profit, and it seeks to explain "the cultural fit between shared fictions about the body and the reducing methods of the era."[25] Schwartz consistently marshals the familiar rhetoric of historical materialism, casting diets as superstructural reflections of the internal contradictions of late capitalism: the dietary emphasis on abstinence and fasting at the opening of the century corresponds to an economic stage of "primitive accumulation" where wealth is a function of saving; when markets expand and increase the importance of distributive technologies, diets turn to a focus on metabolism; in the era of industrial manufacture, people count calories; in a Keynesian era of massaging markets, attention turns to appetite; in an age of capitalist monopoly, dieters are terrified into participation by rumors of heart attacks and diabetes; and when markets have reached their extensive and intensive limits, diets turn to fitness, "capitalism's last hope" in order to accommodate greater consumption and displace the looming crisis of overproduction.[26]

In reading diet trends as neither incidental nor progressive, but rather as symptomatic of distinct prescientific assumptions and economic demands, Schwartz's approach is similar to my own. Nevertheless, his narrative is unsatisfying for at least two reasons: first, it is too "local," as if historical materialism were effective at explaining minor cultural variations instead of broad historical movements; second, Schwartz's facts seem odd, since it is peculiar to say the least to identify the early twentieth century with an age of "primitive accumulation" where wealth is a function of savings (Marx debunked this idea in 1867), and since it is difficult in retrospect to imagine why Schwartz thought markets had reached their extensive and intensive limits in 1986.

Nonetheless, I appreciate the move and, as will become clear, even borrow from it significantly. But rather than identify these five dubious periods of diet, I see three diet paradigms in the twentieth century. The first stage of twentieth-century American dieting, what I will call the metabolic stage, arises from an application of industrial logic to discourses of human health and medicine. In this paradigm, the human body is conceived as a machine, susceptible to the same pathologies of fatigue and breakdown as other machines and with a demonstrable, calculable equivalence between inputs and outputs. In the United States, this approach is inaugurated by Wilbur Atwater, who spent the 1880s demonstrating this equivalence in the human body by putting subjects in a chamber— a calorimeter—in order to precisely measure the inputs (food, drink, and oxygen) and outputs (excreta, carbon dioxide, and heat) and to demonstrate that energy is neither created nor destroyed in the human body. [27] This strict, mechanical approach to diet treats the body as a machine and recommends finding the diet that offers the precise amount of energy necessary to keep it moving efficiently without overwhelming it with surplus. Atwater evokes the elective affinity between this approach to diet and industrial approaches to labor, calling it a "pecuniary economy of food" that sought to maximize "human cost and efficiency."[28] At this point, food is approached not as substance to be engaged ethically and qualitatively, but as an economic resource to be engaged quantitatively.

This model would be picked up in the early twentieth century by noted economist, social reformer, and (therefore) eugenicist Irving Fisher, the first to advise Americans to measure their food not by "weight or bulk" but instead by how much energy they contain, as measured in calories.[29] Fisher calls calories "fuel units" or "food value," providing a model of individual metabolism directly analogous to Marxist economics in which value is measure of energy stored in a commodity.[30] The book containing this advice, *How to Live*, was first published in 1915, and by 1918 it was in its fifteenth edition and carrying an enthusiastic preface from ex-president William Howard Taft, who had recently lost seventy pounds by counting calories. Also in 1918, what has been called America's first diet best seller, Lulu Hunt Peters's *Diet and Health: With Key to the Calories*, "dedicated by permission to Herbert Hoover," hit the shelves offering the same advice: "Instead of saying one slice of bread, or a piece of pie, you will say 100 calories of bread, 350 calories of pie."[31] Making the pecuniary model only slightly more explicit, Peters states, "In war time it is a crime to hoard food . . . Yet there are hundreds of thousands of individuals all over America who are hoarding food . . . *They have vast amounts of this valuable commodity stored away in their own anatomy.*"[32]

As Schwartz points out, if counting calories did not work, the only real alternative for those seeking to lose weight in this period was to boost the body's metabolism, either by raising the heart rate or by accelerating the passage of food through the digestive tract.[33] Dinitrophenol, a compound that works by raising the taker's metabolism by as much as 50 percent, was a wildly popular prescription for promoting weight loss until it was suppressed in 1938.[34] The other popular prescription was for diuretics, which promised to flush ingested material through the body rather than let it settle in as increased body mass. The rhythms and technologies of industrial production provide the model and the vocabulary for metabolically focused diet programs; just as the road to industrial success is to increase the rate of production, the road to dietary health was to increase the rate of metabolism. This model is on clear display from the diet gurus of the day, from Horace Fletcher ("The Great Masticator") who insisted on using the right tools (the teeth, rather than the stomach) to prepare foods for absorption, to Fletcher's disciple John Harvey Kellogg and Kellogg's cross-town rival Charles W. Post, both of whom promised to cure all manner of industrial maladies (from obesity to anxiety to depression) by regulating metabolism. Kellogg and Post shared a goal of developing efficient foods that could pass through the human digestive system, leaving behind as many nutrients as possible without obstructing an ideally frictionless process of absorption. For Kellogg, this meant a progressive vegetarian diet (starting with nothing but grapes and proceeding up to grains such as his brother William's invention, the corn flake) and an enthusiastic condemnation of the human energies wasted in sexual activity.[35]

While gluttony and obesity had been condemned on moral grounds for centuries, it was not typically characterized as a health issue, nor did it inspire mass participation in intentional programs of weight loss, until after 1900.[36] Ideals of slenderness after 1900 were largely targeted at women's bodies; corpulence remained a sign of status among men while slenderness became a mark of class privilege among women in this period.[37] Fisher's and Peters's books, however, were not aimed at women but at the general population increasingly concerned about losing weight. Turner has identified at least two reasons for this new obsession.[38] First, and perhaps most obviously, the United States in 1918 had tremendous demand for healthy bodies to staff both the growing labor force and the rapidly growing military gearing up for World War I. The pull of diet, as evidenced by the previous Peters quote indicating a homology between the individual body and the body politic, suggests that physical fitness became both a medical possibility and a national duty, thus participating in the normalization and control of "the population" that emerged as the purview of the state in the liberal era.[39] Second, and less obviously, American society in this period was also seeing rapid development of fixed-space public accommodations and commodities, from restaurants and movie theaters to mass-manufactured clothing and furniture, that were increasingly modeled on a standardized body type. It became increasingly inconvenient, in other words, to be fat.

Together, these dynamics reveal a discourse of diet slightly different than the one identified by Schwartz. Rather than a superstructural reflection of the demands of "Late Capitalism," the discourse of diet functions here as a technology of population management, promoting ideals of nationalism and self-discipline that are essential to producing subjects willing and able to aid the national interest both militarily and economically. Further, it produces a mass of standardized bodies with predictable demands and abilities, essential to the smooth functioning and steady growth of an industrial economy, while also generating a vast bank of data about human bodies—about needs, desires, and abilities, illness, and mortality—that will better allow for predictable institutions of social order and the health of the nation.

Both scientific and popular discourses of diet in this period were beholden to the language of the thermodynamics and the metaphorics of industrial production. In this straightforward industrial diet, excessive girth represented energy unpatriotically hoarded, and the key to weight loss was invariably to either slow the intake or accelerate the output of that energy. The body is a machine that burns fuel, wears out, and can be manipulated to move faster or slower, and weight loss is achieved through a paradigm of industrial standardization and productive efficiency. Health of individual bodies and bodies politic were subject to the same threats: entropy, fatigue, and the development of so-called dead weight.

This industrial model perhaps seems simple and intuitive enough, and the simple refrain "count your calories" might still seem to resonate with dietary advice a century later. But this metabolic approach to diet largely fell out of favor after the Great Depression when a new paradigm that would dominate dietary advice for the bulk of the twentieth century came into fashion. In this new paradigm, weight control was pursued much less through manipulating metabolism than through managing desire and promoting individual self-control. Overweight bodies were diagnosed with faulty desires, not slow metabolisms, and the key to weight loss was appetite control and will power. Out with dinitrophenol and diuretics; in with appetite suppressants and psychological treatments of compulsive eating.

Though amphetamines had been on the market since 1932 as treatment for asthma, depression, and anxiety (as well as for recreation, of course), they were first considered as a diet aid in 1938, the same year dinitrophenol was taken off the market.[40] By 1970, perhaps 10 billion tabs of Benzedrine, the amphetamine of choice, were being prescribed annually—at least 2 billion of which were for weight loss.[41] Crucially, the logic behind prescribing amphetamines (a.k.a. "speed") was never to boost metabolism, but to suppress appetite. Over the years, such standardbearing, over-the-counter appetite suppressants such as Dexatrim and Accutrim have been made with amphetamines—originally phenylpropanolamine (banned by the U.S. Food and Drug Administration [FDA] in 2000 for its link to strokes) and then ephedrine (now controversial for its easy conversion into crystal methamphetamine).[42] This period also saw a proliferation of "high satiety" diets designed to trick the body into feeling full, and the aforementioned proliferation of diet sodas and light beer that would allow people to indulge without gaining weight.

More dramatically, however, this is the period when weight first got classified as a psychological issue. An influential study in the *Journal of the American Medical Association* traced obesity to emotional problems like anxiety and insecurity in 1947.[43] That same year, *Time Magazine* profiled Hilde Bruch (who would eventually introduce Americans to eating disorders like anorexia and bulimia) for claiming that weight problems stem from "low self-esteem" and a sense of "helplessness."[44] In 1952, *Newsweek* profiled "The Fat Personality," and by 1959, *The New York Times Magazine* was reporting that 90 percent of obesity was "psychogenic" in nature.[45] Bruch's *Eating Disorders* gave the definitive statement of psychology and diet in 1973, but the emotional approach to diet reached its political apotheosis in Susie Orbach's instant classic from 1978, *Fat Is a Feminist Issue*, in which biological theories of weight gain were summarily rejected with her claim that the primary reason women get fat is emotional disturbance stemming from patriarchal domination.[46]

The bellwether of the psychological paradigm, however, is the rise in support groups designed to help people lose weight. By far the most successful of these endeavors is Weight Watchers, founded in 1962 by self-described "Formerly Fat Housewife" Jean Nidetch after she lost 72 pounds by following a diet developed by New York public health doctor Norman Joliffe to treat cardiac health. In her official account of the business, Nidetch explains that she founded Weight Watchers as a support group where overweight women (and a few men) could come to talk about compulsive eating and offer mutual support to provide the intestinal fortitude to overcome this compulsion with will power.[47] Though Nidetch insists that dieters must follow Joliffe's diet "to the letter," the diet itself is all but irrelevant to the Weight Watchers business plan. Indeed, Weight Watchers neither owns nor sells the diet itself (Nidetch admits it is freely available from the New York Department of Health), nor does the Weight Watchers literature endeavor to explain it. What Weight Watchers offers is emotional support: "Actually, what's been added to Dr. Joliffe's diet is talk, it's really not much more than talk."[48] Though Joliffe's diet is quite detailed and inflexible—the rules include eating three servings of fruit per day, five servings of fish per week, and, perhaps most curiously, "[y]ou must eat liver once per week"[49]—Weight Watchers consistently appeals to a psychological rather than a metabolic paradigm, diagnosing the overweight body as defective in its desires rather than its metabolism. For Nidetch, the benefits of losing weight are similarly psychological: being able to buy more attractive clothing, feeling good about oneself, and being "in control" of oneself.[50] The business trades in a rhetoric of personal empowerment rather than industrial efficiency:

"Empathy, rapport, and mutual understanding are the keys."[51] Clearly, the idea is that women (and some men) are constitutionally ill-equipped for the industrial age.

Like the metabolic paradigm, the psychological paradigm can be read as a symptom of broader currents of politics and economics. Peter Stearns notes that after the Depression, inefficiency and scarcity largely ceased to be defining problems in American society. In the so-called affluent society, as productivity soared and credit became widely available, the threat to the health of the nation was no longer fatigue but a depleted moral fiber stemming from rampant consumerism.[52] Schwartz links the new-found suspicion of individual appetite to a Keynesian suspicion about self-regulating markets; while the medical and dietary establishment had previously conceded that hunger is a reliable guide of caloric need, there was now growing suspicion of the body and individual desire: "The body, like the economy after 1929, could not be trusted to regulate itself."[53]

These explanations trace a paradigm shift to specific changes in social and political order after an economic collapse. But they curiously refrain from linking them to a more dramatic shift in U.S. political economy from an industrial to a service economy. It is easy enough to characterize Weight Watchers as a paradigmatic success story in the service economy: the official Weight Watchers literature regularly casts Nidetch in the familiar Horatio Alger narrative in recognizably populist themes, and while Weight Watchers does sell some tangible products like cookbooks and packaged meals, the program's success came from selling a service—emotional support. Reading Corey Robin's commanding study of political fear, it becomes clear that Weight Watchers is no mere service provider, but is a provider of the service that responds to the dominant concerns permeating U.S. culture in the years after World War II.[54] Robin notes that the distinctive political fear of this era was neither death at the hands of a violent enemy nor the poverty and desperation memorable from the 1930s, but rather erasure of the individual by technologies of totalitarianism. Despite the immediate memory of the Depression, war, and the Holocaust, the defining political texts of the day focused much less on mass slaughter and much more on the erasure of individual will. This is the case in George Orwell's *1984* (1949), in which dystopia inheres in an absence of individual thought; Hannah Arendt's *The Origins of Totalitarianism* (1951), in which the author prepares the reader for the possibility that dictatorship is an inevitable part of modernity; and then her *Eichmann in Jerusalem* (1963), in which the atrocities of the Holocaust are cast as the work of a minor bureaucrat. Alongside Theodor Adorno et al.'s *The Authoritarian Personality* (1950) and Herbert Marcuse's *One-Dimensional Man* (1964), Stanley Milgram's studies of conformity (1961), and pop sociologies like David Riesman's *The Lonely Crowd* (1953), Sloan Wilson's *Man in the Gray Flannel Suit* (1955), and William H. Whyte's *The Organization Man* (1956), one gets the picture of a society increasingly anxious over the maintenance of individual will in the face of state power, media indoctrination, or the corporate business structure.

In other words, will power is not just the key to weight loss in this period; it is the response to the threat of totalitarian society, and the key to success in the gentler, consumer, mass society. Kandi Stinson and Robert Putnam thus see Weight Watchers—along with organizations such as Overeaters Anonymous (est. 1958), Weight Losers Institute (est. 1968), Diet Center (est. 1971), NutriSystem (est. 1971), and Jenny Craig (est. 1983)—as a branch of a self-help and support group culture that flourished in the United States from the 1950s through the 1990s.[55] Typically, these groups emphasize the healing power of bringing private concerns into public view and offer both solace and legitimacy to populations otherwise lacking in social capital.[56] As Heyes notes, self-awareness, self-confidence, and self-control are the overriding themes of organizations like Weight Watchers. Like so many other participants in this culture of self-improvement, Weight Watchers offers the kind of individual empowerment seemingly being threatened by so many institutions of late capitalism.[57]

Eventually, the use of appetite suppressants and group therapy would fall out of favor in the American dietary discourse to be replaced with a wholly new understanding of why bodies gain weight. Critser has chronicled a new era of dietary permissiveness starting in the 1990s, when a slew of diet books abandoned the familiar dietary mantras about self-restraint and argued that it was possible to lose weight while still eating "all you want."[58] The most visible champion of this new paradigm would be Robert Atkins, the physician who successfully changed that narrative of American dietary discourse away from appetite and toward the role of hormones in regulating weight.[59] Along with other hormone-based diets like the Zone and South Beach, Atkins defined a dietary Zeitgeist that lasted (at least) through the next decade.[60]

The logic behind the Atkins diet is that consuming carbohydrates causes the body to accelerate its production of insulin, the hormone that tells the body to convert dietary sugar to fat, and this acceleration, in turn, leads to heightened hunger. From within this hormonal paradigm, overweight bodies are not seen as inefficient machines nor as emotionally disturbed consumers, but as transmitters of bad data. The key to weight loss in the hormonal paradigm is not consuming fewer calories or managing your appetite, but in regulating the messages that the brain receives from the food you consume; you can eat all you want so long as your body does not get the message to store what it receives. Gone is the counting of calories and the guilt of overindulgence. Instead, the new paradigm promises dietary success through the successful management of information.

It has become quite commonplace to note how the centrality of communication, data, and digital commodities in the Internet age has disrupted the most familiar metrics of value inherited from generations past. As Mark Poster summarily puts this, capitalism's organization around "[s]team energy, wage labor, and heavy machinery" gave way to a more expansive focus on "consumption, fantasy, and desire" in midcentury, a regime that was itself eclipsed by the trade in "symbols, sounds, and images."[61] Indeed, the proliferation of digital commodities disrupts the assumptions of both classical political economy (which roots value in supply and demand) and Marxist political economy (which roots value in labor), since digital commodities are infinitely replicable with minimal human labor or material resources. In our current information economy, neither the efficient production of goods nor the effective management of desire is necessary to realize profits; stock prices rise and fall with little to no relation to productivity or even revenues. Fredric Jameson and David Harvey point to the end of the global gold standard as precipitating this new kind of postmodern economy, though the boundless optimism of recent tech and real estate bubbles also depended on a decoupling of economics from thermodynamic assumptions about value.[62] In this situation, diet paradigms modeled on thermodynamics and restraint became similarly anachronistic: if we can get rich by controlling information, why can't we get thin the same way?

If it seems as if my identification of paradigm shifts from production to distribution to communication is too obviously an attempt to identify a shift in economic significance from industrial manufacturing plants to retail outlets to the Internet (from industrial to a service to an information economy), note that the shift to an emphasis on hormones marks a dramatic shift from the thermodynamic insights about scarcity and consumption that governed economic activity for a century. That is, hormones neither produce matter nor coordinate its movement, but communicate messages to various organs that are themselves involved in metabolism. The dominant approach to diet in both scientific and popular literature over the past decade has not been to maximize efficiency or to manage demand, but to control the information; it is neither Fordist nor Keynesian, but properly financial. The control of information as profit provides the ideology that justifies hormonal approaches to diet. Atkins is the information diet for the information age.

Diet as Ideology

In the paradigm shifts just chronicled, the issue is not whether one approach rather than another effectively facilitates weight loss; restricting calories, suppressing appetite, and avoiding carbohydrates are all viable strategies for losing weight. These paradigms did not shift when one approach was revealed as defective, but when an alternative vocabulary and set of assumptions proved more satisfying as explanations for the operations of the human body. This is consistent with Kuhn's narrative, in which the scientific revolutions owe less to a progressive move toward truth than to a changing set of hegemonic assumptions. But what Kuhn does not address is the sociological explanations for *why* some assumptions become popular. Marx does this when he explains why alienating religions become hegemonic under the conditions of alienated labor— that is, for Marx, ideology *works* when it corresponds to peoples' daily experiences.[63] Similarly, Weber also does this by explaining how Calvinism and capitalism had an elective affinity such that they could reinforce and amplify their shared assumptions about industriousness and success. In short, there is something about the organization of the world (say, economic or political impotence) that would render a deterministic explanation of the universe appealing and other organizations (say, one of upward mobility and consumer freedom) that would give credence to narratives of free will. The point, in other words, is not that either of these explanations is "right" or "wrong," but that they are, in varying conditions, satisfying or unsatisfying. As Kuhn puts it, "neither proof nor error is at issue."[64] So the question is not, "Which is right?" but rather, "Why believe one rather than the other?"

The story of Atkins is particularly revealing in this regard. Robert Atkins first published *Dr. Atkins' Diet Revolution* in 1972, and though it immediately turned heads with its counterintuitive argument that regulating hormones would allow us to weigh less and eat more, it did not inspire the diet revolution that he (and his publishers) clearly expected. Like Copernicus, Atkins was quickly branded a heretic for challenging the orthodoxy that governed his field, and nearly every other doctor on the planet was warning that his advice was quite dangerous. Atkins released a sequel, *Dr. Atkins's New Diet Revolution* in 1992, again to impressive sales but still just as much skepticism. Five years later, however, *Science* was reporting that studies of obesity and weight loss were "dominated" by talk of hormones,[65] and by 2003, thanks largely to a controversial story by *New York Times* science writer Gary Taubes, Atkins was a household name and popular restaurant chains like Applebee's were developing special menus to accommodate what critics called an epidemic of "carbophobia."[66] What's more, the specific logic of a low-carb diet dates back at least 150 years: William Banting recommended this approach to weight loss in the 1860s, soon after which Americans referred to the activity as "banting" rather than "dieting."[67] Schwartz identifies a series of specific, distinct, and fairly popular low-carb high-fat diet fads in the 1880s, 1940s, 1950s, and 1960s.[68] In other words, Atkins's book had been on shelves for thirty years, and his ideas had been in circulation for over a century before scientists and dieters quite suddenly decided he was right.

Of course, there may be very crude and immediate material reasons for the popularity of Atkins around 2000. In the previous forty years, the yield from U.S. farms had increased by some 500 calories per person per day;[69] in this situation of caloric abundance, ascetic diets predicated on self-denial are both difficult to market and a macroeconomic liability. Further, the American cuisine became steadily richer in carbohydrates through the 1980s, as the "low-fat" foods that came to fill supermarket shelves were largely produced by replacing fat with carbohydrates.[70] Cutting carbs, in other words, is a more viable diet option when carbs are a heftier proportion of your diet. Atkins also requires consuming a lot of high-protein, low-carb foods, especially meat. But meat was very expensive in the early 1970s, and it is only with the persistent support of agricultural subsidies (starting with the Nixon administration) that it has become economically feasible (even cheap) to eat meat at every meal. Finally, the rhetoric of the Atkins "revolution" resonates with an increasingly permissive culture and a revamped approach to indulgence and entitlement indulgence through the Reagan years,[71] while its populist rejection of the official dietary advice capitalizes on increasing skepticism about government and scientific expertise.[72]

But more fundamentally, it is difficult to imagine widespread support for the idea that the body is governed by messages—rather than matter, energy, or will—before our transition into an era in which the economy itself is organized around the trade of information. Whereas a metabolic diet has an elective affinity with an industrial economy and a psychological diet resonated with a service economy, a hormonal diet has an elective affinity with an information economy. Again, low-carb diets are not new; what *is* new, apparently, is a widespread comfort with the idea that hormones govern weight. The hormonal paradigm, freely circulating but largely derided for over a century, did not become a candidate for dietary commonsense until this explanation of the human body (like psychological and metabolic explanations that preceded it) conformed to established strategies for producing, distributing, and accumulating value. Biologically, low-carb diets have worked for a long time; politically, they only started working with the rise of the Internet.

Weight Watchers's accommodation to this new paradigm is equally revealing. Since its founding, the business has gone through various changes in ownership and strategy, though it has remained by far the most successful enterprise in the commercial weight loss industry. Before the business went public in 2001, it developed a lucrative brand of packaged foods and revised the Joliffe diet multiple times before scrapping it entirely in 1997 for its trademark Points program, which uses a specific formula to help dieters manage their weight by balancing their calories against a "penalty" for dietary fat and a "bonus" for eating fiber. Though Weight Watchers remains steadfast in its commitment to the psychological paradigm, as some one million clients still visit support group meetings each week, the rhetoric of Weight Watchers since the mid-1990s has gradually shifted away from telling dieters what they "must" or "must not" eat to a greater emphasis on "individual freedom" and "personal choice."[73] Indeed, Points is now the face of the brand and is marketed, like Atkins, under the banner of letting dieters eat whatever they want (so long as they do not exceed a prescribed number of points per day).

These rhetorical and strategic shifts are notable for a few reasons. First, because Nidetch was famously vocal that there was nothing proprietary about Weight Watchers; the business never sold dietary advice and all she contributed, she maintained, was the idea that women should support one another: "[I]t's really not much more than talk."[74] In the past ten years, however, Weight Watchers has floundered through intellectual property law, marketing Points as a brand but being unable to protect the formula (since formulas are not eligible for patent protection). While the business still *sells* a service, what they *market* is software. This shift is also notable because as public attention turned to carbs, Weight Watchers produced more and more literature about hormones. But their argument has not been that hormones are important for how they affect blood sugar, but for how they affect mood and appetite.[75] In other words, Weight Watchers appropriated the new language (hormones) without abandoning the old paradigm (psychology). But finally, this shift is notable because in 2010, Weight Watchers overhauled the Points formula to keep up with what they called "the latest science." While the program had, for a decade, been organized around a balance of calories, fat, and fiber, the new program makes no mention of calories; they have been replaced by protein and carbohydrates.[76] Welcome to the new paradigm.

The Biggest Loser

Histories of diet are typically organized around a presumed irony that, as Americans grew more interested in dieting over the twentieth century, they also grew more overweight.[77] Assuming this correlation is accurate, it only appears *ironic* if we believe that more attention to dieting should cause lower body weights. If, however, we consider that Americans grew more interested in dieting *because* they were growing more overweight, or that Americans grew more interested in dieting because of a cultural demand for entrepreneurial, disciplined, and self-regulating subjects, then this relationship looks less *ironic* than it does *ideological* and *biopolitical*. The intensification of diet—both in its transformation from a feminized and medicalized discourse to a generalized and ubiquitous one and in its transformation from an industrial model aimed at individual bodies to a hormonal one aimed at the minutest level of biochemical regulation—affords individuals both the tools and the motivation for increasing levels of self-governance. It produces, in other words, the very subjects appropriate to neoliberal order.

The shifts chronicled in this chapter do not correspond to a steady march toward a greater truth about the human body, but they do deploy ever more sophisticated and intensive forms of surveillance, while offering ideological cover against the anxieties of that surveillance. While the medical interventions of Atwater, Kellogg, and Post conform to the kind of disciplinary activities endemic to hospitals and prisons as described by Foucault in *Discipline and Punish*, Weight Watchers removes that technique from the fixed confines of a hospital or calorimeter, assigning to each individual the responsibility for monitoring and measuring their body's activities (not only eating and exercise but also their cravings and desires) as a matter of habit. Dieters on Atkins need not monitor and restrict their desire to consume as they do on Weight Watchers, but they must attend to the messages sent by their brain to their pancreas, paying constant attention to the forces and substances that allow their bodies to succeed or fail. What unites these paradigms is a promise of self-control in a world of steadily declining agency, where it is threatened first by industrial technology, then by mass media and totalitarian politics, and finally by collections of financial resources and information databases used for niche marketing and consumer manipulation.

While crusaders like Nidetch might seem to offer political displacement in promising women a sense of empowerment that only distracts from the obstacles to realizing the liberal promise of political and economic power, Heyes and Cruikshank convincingly argue that they also offer real strategies for responding to real threats to political and economic powerlessness. The tools of self-construction and self-control afforded by Weight Watchers, for instance, do, in fact, allow individuals to exercise the kind of self-awareness and discipline required for any kind of belief in (and therefore exercise of) individual sovereignty. As Cruikshank puts this, self-help literature "does not so much avoid 'real' political problems as transform the level on which it is possible to address those problems."[78] Heyes and Cruikshank thus resist the diet as a form of subjectification (and thus the crude victim narratives from the likes of Orbach and Bruch), emphasizing instead the productive power dieting culture. The discourse and practice of dieting, they argue, produces the kind of self-monitoring and self-reliant subjects that are indeed prepared for success in global capitalism. That is, it is not just false consciousness that Weight Watchers promotes by telling people they can be "in control" of themselves (though there is this, since, it seems clear that the kind of self-control promoted by Nidetch is less about democracy and more about self-esteem); such "practices of the self" also produce the kind of entrepreneurial subjects that are required and rewarded by capitalist markets.

In this light, the politics of dieting is profoundly ambivalent. On the one hand, it participates fully in the politics of individual responsibility, where complicated nexus of the availability of food, exercise, and health care are displaced onto the idea that individuals have the responsibility to care for their own bodies, while simultaneously producing the kind of predictable and knowable bodies that can be calculated, measured, and planned for by actuaries and health care providers. On the other, the "care of the self" does produce in subjects a kind of agency and entitlement that is essential to successful participation in democratic culture and economic markets. In this sense, the metamorphosis of diet literature away from such crude, authoritarian proclamations about what you must or must not eat, and toward regimes that place on the individual the ultimate responsibility for deciding what to eat, *is* a narrative of individual empowerment. Narratives of diet respond directly to anxieties about individual sovereignty and offer tools for protecting that sovereignty, which ironically advocate taking more responsibility for our own health, productivity, and ultimately smooth incorporation into the predictable networks of global capital. What could be more ideological than that?

2   EATING ALONE

WHILE SO MUCH DISCUSSION OF food in the United States is couched in the individualistic language of choice and self-control, characterizations of food as a private or personal issue stand in stark contrast with the anthropological and sociological literatures on the role of food in establishing regional or national culture. Food historian Margaret Visser notes this paradox, and the tendency of food to conflate facile separations of public and private, noting how in rituals of shared eating from family dinners to religious feasts "satisfaction of the most individual of needs becomes a means of creating community."[1] Of course, cultural critics since World War II have indicted the American food system—the developments of fast food and TV dinners and the consequent decline in family meals—in their lamentations of lost community and cultural decline. But these nostalgic visions of collective eating tend to offer technological explanations for our mode of eating and ignore a larger issue: they point to industrial processes that made it both possible and expedient to eat alone, though they have no explanation for why it would be *desirable*—why the celebration and pleasure of eating together would succumb to the convenience and pragmatism of eating alone.

In this chapter, I aim to correct this neglect by rooting the privatization of food not to any technological or economic developments of the twentieth century but to scientific, political, economic, and aesthetic developments of the seventeenth century. In short, I argue that while transformations of the twentieth century made it convenient to eat alone, transformations of the seventeenth century made it desirable. Far before the putative moral and communal breakdown typically associated with the late twentieth century, the trend toward eating alone started in the transformation of social order at the end of the Middle Ages. In this transformation, one sees the practice and representation of eating removed from public life. Eating became a private engagement with the democratization of private dining areas, a decline in public festivals organized around meals, and a dramatic rise in taboos against recognition of digestive processes. The privatization of food, I argue, owes to the increased importance of industrial technologies and capitalist markets, a shift also evident in the organic "body politic" giving way to the legalistic "social contract" as the organizing metaphor of political life.

This shift can be inferred from expressions and valences in scientific, political, and aesthetic treatises of the day. Together, these texts help construct a set of cultural values that privatize food. That is, while Locke's *Second Treatise* and Hobbes's *Leviathan* do not offer explicit treatments of how we do or should eat, they provide ways of thinking about selves and identity that become widely accepted and have specific implications for understanding what it means to eat. Further, looking at what these texts do (or do not) have to say about eating reveals a particular understanding of what it is to be a human being, an understanding that has significant implications for the establishment of epistemological, aesthetic, and political value.

From Bodies Politic to Political Bodies

Though romantics of various stripes have described a decline in social capital and family bonds since World War II by tracing the demise of civic groups, family meals, or bowling leagues, political theorists have identified a profound (and roughly parallel) shift in Western civilization in the sixteenth and seventeenth centuries. This period of transition from the Middle Ages to the modern era saw a rising importance of private space at the expense of public life.[2] The extension of religious tolerance, representative government, and capitalist markets—the institutions of modern liberalism—are by now well rehearsed. What is less well rehearsed is how the enclosures of land and the privatization of space entailed a privatization of bodily functions, with both legal and social codes growing intolerant of public recognition of the metabolic operations of the human body. This period saw a vast proliferation of norms governing eating habits, laws privatizing bodily wastes, and taboos against bodily functions. Before the changing representations of the human body discussed in the previous chapter, one can see dramatic changes in political, medical, and aesthetic representations of the body's relation to other bodies in this period, changes that correspond to and reinforce the demands of a liberal discourse of human autonomy and personal responsibility. Liberal society did not merely privatize space, consciousness, and economic activity; it also pushed into a private sphere the operations associated with the material maintenance of the human body. The body politic grew intolerant of an unwieldy and increasingly disgusting human body.

The biological body figures prominently in the history of political thought. The notion that a political community shares the organic and harmonious organization of the biological body has long been captured with the familiar metaphor of a body politic—a metaphor as old as recorded political thought itself. In its earliest appearances, the metaphor evoked a harmonious political community in which each of the members had an organic connection to one another and to the body as a whole—each essential to the health operations of the society and, perhaps more important, each incapable of surviving on their own. Though certainly not the first, John of Salisbury's twelfth-century articulation is among the favorites: "The position of the head in the republic is occupied . . . by a prince. . . . The place of the heart is occupied by the senate. . . . The duties of the ears, eyes, and mouth are claimed by the judges and governors of provinces. . . . The hands coincide with the officials and soldiers . . . [etc.]."[3]

As David Hale has pointed out, this conception of mutual dependence and primal unity, this notion that individuals are but organs in a broader political body rather than self-determining and rights-bearing agents, lost tremendous favor in the transition out of the Middle Ages.[4] While the metaphor of a body politic of course endured, it lost its metaphysical significance around 1649, when the English body politic cut off its own head by executing Charles I. Hereafter, the metaphor referred less to an organic unity of the people than to the legal apparatus of the state.

Surely because the metaphysical connotations of a body politic no longer resonated with the transforming political landscape of modern liberalism, the metaphor surrendered its position at the center of political discourse and was quickly and summarily replaced by an alternative guiding political metaphor: the social contract. Representation of society as a legal arrangement instead of an organism—a contract instead of a body—suggested that society was made up of autonomous individuals who would *choose* how and where to join public life. Hereafter, participation in public life would be voluntary and intentional rather than organic and metaphysical; individuals are now by convention and choice part of a social unit, and they are completely capable of divorcing from that society should they want. This shift is not merely rhetorical. The replacement of the organic metaphor of a body with the legal metaphor of a contract conveys a profound metaphysical shift as well—from a worldview predicated on unity, dependence, and organic connections to one predicated on autonomy, individual choice, and legal obligation.[5]

Tellingly, this period saw not only an increasing distrust of metaphysical baggage of the biological metaphor but also of the material operations of actual bodies. In Norbert Elias's canonical study of what he calls "the civilizing process," the sixteenth and seventeenth centuries display a retreat of bodily functions into a secluded private realm, as European civilization developed all manner of social taboos and manners concerning "outward bodily propriety"—not only posture, gestures, and table manners but also the appropriate way to deal with snot, saliva, and vomit; how to handle food and feces; when and how to pick your teeth, wash your hands, or chew your food; and the acceptability of coughing, farting, and sneezing.[6] Arguing that a society's level of "civilization" can be measured by the number of these things that are done in private, Elias shows how codes of conduct that were relatively stable for centuries underwent rapid change in this period, as thresholds for embarrassment were lowered and more and more functions were "properly" relegated to a private space.[7] Further, he shows how formerly common and totally acceptable practices (say, blowing your nose into your hand or spitting out a disagreeable piece of food) were at first explicitly condemned and then quite quickly became unmentionable; it became rude not merely to release these substances in public but to even mention the existence of snot, saliva, or gas. Summarily, while the Middle Ages had no shortage of rules and customs defining proper behavior,

> [w]hat was lacking . . . was the invisible wall of affects which seems now to rise between one human body and another, repelling and separating, the wall which is often perceptible today at the mere approach of something that has been in contact with the mouth or hands of someone else, and which manifests itself as embarrassment at the mere sight of many bodily functions to others, and often at their mere mention, or as a feeling

of shame when one's own functions are exposed to the gaze of others, and by no means only then.[8]

This "invisible wall of affects" at least partly explains, for Elias, why "[e]ating and drinking [in the Middle Ages] occupied a far more central position in social life than today."[9] The modern protocols of eating and digestion (from not talking with your mouth full to renouncing scatological humor) are designed to conceal the inevitable and prosaic breach of this wall that separates the self from the world—a wall that is anathema to the logic of a body politic but essential to that of a social contract. As Elspeth Probyn notes, the simple mechanics of digestion compromise the line between bodies: "[F]ood goes in, and then, broken down, it comes out of the body, and every time this happens our bodies are affected."[10] With the outside world fusing with the self (ingestion) and pieces of the self being deposited into the hand, tablecloth, or toilet (excretion), the process of digestion "question[s] bodies and identities."[11]

Elias claims that "the whole process of what we call civilization is the movement of segregation, this hiding 'behind the scenes' of what has become distasteful."[12] And what has become distasteful, he continues, is recognition of our animality, our mortality, and our vulnerability— features of the human condition that are on vivid display in the mechanics of digestion and metabolism, as the external world enters and mixes with the body.[13] The civilizing process, in other words, involves the privatization of animal nature and material life, as public life becomes less tolerant of the concerns of the body and more focused on the refined sensibilities of the mind. Though we remain no different from beasts when we are having bowel movements or devouring the flesh of slaughtered animals, we are civilized to the extent that we subordinate that desire and that practice to a calculated system of rules, manners, and spaces.

Mikhail Bakhtin makes this very same argument in contrasting the public celebrations of the body in festivals and carnivals endemic to the Middle Ages with the more sterile, domesticated, and privatized feasts of the modern era, as "[t]he carnival spirit . . . was gradually transformed into a mere holiday mood."[14] Specifically, Bakhtin identifies a premodern worldview in which bodily orifices (in particular, the mouth and the anus—that is, the opposite ends of the gastrointestinal tract) signified an openness to the ostensibly external world, an openness that was celebrated in public acts of consumption and incorporation. Premodern celebrations, he explains, called attention to the vulnerability of the individual body to the material environment, taking great pleasure in the experience and representation of gastrointestinal processes that blurred the boundaries between the self and the other. The "grotesque body" celebrates its openness, and so "the act of eating is joyful, triumphant."[15] Bakhtin contrasts this with a modern view of the body, in which orifices are sites of weakness and anxiety—sites of a loss of integrity and the failure to distinguish the self. In modern representations of the body, this openness is hidden, privatized, and even psychologized; it becomes a point of shame and reminder of mortality.[16] Flatulence and bowel movements, for example, passed from being central components in popular discourse and folk humor during the Middle Ages into crude topics mentioned only in the lowest of lowbrow culture. Though "the bodily lower stratum" once figured prominently in public discourse, modern representations of the orifices and functions of the body "have radically changed their meaning: they have been transferred to the private and psychological level where their connotation becomes narrow and specific, torn away from the direct relation to the life of society and to the cosmic whole."[17]

Whereas the premodern carnival celebrated and enacted the body politic by calling attention to the bounty and incorporation that is collective life, the modern holiday sanitizes the experience, removing it to the private space of the home. Desire and animality are not eliminated, but they are domesticated and subjected to rational control. In public space—the space of politics and collective living—the body comports itself as the rational, autonomous, and discrete being consistent with the metaphor of a social contract.

Of course, eating is but one of the activities coming under scrutiny in this period, and when considering the other processes being written out of public life at the time (such as defecating, vomiting, and nose-picking), the inclination is typically to chalk it up to basic issues of hygiene or primal disgust. But Elias explicitly rejects the notion that these proscriptions are rooted in hygiene since so many of these new codes (e.g., burping at the table or talking with your mouth full, not serving animals with the face attached, or preferring forks to spoons) have nothing whatsoever to do with cleanliness. Even taboos that do seem clearly linked to hygiene are often not—spitting, for instance, became generally distasteful long before people knew that saliva carries germs.[18] Rather, these practices appear to have come into disfavor for the same reason that food became a lesser part of public life: they posed a threat to the idealized representation of the autonomous individual implied by the metaphor of a social contract, announcing the openness and vulnerability of the body right when social order was coming to depend on its boundedness and integrity. As we will see, these ostensibly aesthetic concerns underlie the emergent institutions of bourgeois science, economics, and politics.

The Ontopolitics of Liberalism

Far be it from me to suggest that being civilized means not talking with your mouth full, but the injunction against talking with food in your mouth does seem to be a function of a worldview that is threatened or disoriented by the sight of semichewed food. That is, the decreased tolerance for bodily functions discussed in the previous section corresponds to much larger epistemological, economic, and political developments of the sixteenth and seventeenth centuries. Susan Bordo argues that these developments are exemplified and catalyzed in René Descartes's *Meditations*, which solidified a philosophical transcendence of mind over body. As Descartes announces, "[although] I have a body with which I am very closely united . . . it is certain that this 'I' . . . is entirely . . . distinct from my body."[19]

"The seventeenth century," Bordo bluntly declares, "seems preoccupied with firming the distinction between self and world."[20] Bordo attributes this preoccupation to two distinct sources: First, to Descartes's *Meditations*, in which accurate knowledge depends on a clear separation of the knower from the known. This point (that reliable knowledge demands a critical distance of scientists from their object of study) is now familiar to every college freshman prepared to dismiss as "subjective" or "biased" information not maintaining this distance, and it informs the principle that sound scientific study demands clearly defined spaces (laboratories) in which that distance can be reliably maintained.[21] This priority of "objectivity" also, as Bordo notes, implies the priority of the individual being as the source of both knowledge and value, thus providing the epistemological foundation for a political order organized around individual rights. Second, Bordo argues that the increased importance of machinery and bureaucracy in this period brought along a demand for precise ordering of physical bodies that can be discretely quantified and accurately measured. Industrial production, bureaucratic efficiency, and large-scale commerce demand exact and predictable measurement that requires fixed and stable boundaries around objects; mechanical gears must interact with minimal friction, predictable exchange requires precise calculations of weights and values, and both organizations and machines require that parts can be traded and replaced with minimal disruption to continued operations. Further, with public land being increasingly partitioned into discrete parcels for private use, clear markers of the boundaries between me and not me, between this and that, and between both objects and spaces become increasingly salient. In short, according to Bordo, the border between the self and the other became a site of anxiety in this period precisely because social and economic order was coming to depend on maintaining this border.[22]

This is a period of pervasive "disorientation" and "anxiety," stemming from what Bordo calls a story of the "*parturition* from the organic universe of the Middle Ages and Renaissance, out of which emerged the modern categories of 'self,' 'locatedness,' and 'inwardness.'"[23] In other words, Descartes was reckoning not just with technological innovation and the demand for scientific rigor but with the now familiar challenges to religious and political authorities of the Middle Ages coming by the revolutionary practices and discourses of liberalism. Bordo continues to suggest that the psychoanalytic focus on "separation anxiety" is but the personalized expression of this more general, historical separation of individuals from the earth and from each other. Descartes speaks to this political rather than psychological anxiety by forwarding the value of individual reason, promising both truth and meaning in this condition of individuation. Bordo sees Descartes's insistence that one has either "absolute certainty or epistemological chaos" as a symptom of a broader concern that one has either political authority or social chaos.[24]

Bordo thus offers context to what Elias and Bakhtin say about the increased intolerance for bodily functions in the sixteenth and seventeenth centuries. The substances that cross the border between the self and the other—sweat, excreta, mucous, and especially food—threaten the separation of self from world that is the precondition of knowledge and order. As a result, these substances capture the anxiety about the borders that are becoming increasingly important to maintaining social order, metonymically standing for the various gaps in the foundational myths of liberal subjectivity and capitalist exchange. Bodily fluids that blur or permeate the borders between the self and the other, as well as the activities that call attention to that blurring, call into question the discreteness of bodies—a discreteness that was coming to provide the basis for more and more essential social institutions. Pointing to "hunger, thirst, pain, and so on" as "confused modes of thinking which have their origin in . . . the union and apparent fusion of the mind and the body,"[25] Descartes not only demands that knowers establish a clear barrier between self and world in order to avoid confusion but also establishes the direct counterpoint to the popular wisdom (and materialist mantra) that you are what you eat. Indeed, if you are what you eat, how can you ever separate yourself from the world you are studying? Cogito ergo sum.[26]

This explains why, as Bordo and other feminist philosophers have shown, the seventeenth century inaugurates not only a series of norms regulating the composure and representation of the body but also a set of philosophical narratives that officially neglect the operations of the body. Elizabeth Grosz, for instance, identifies "a profound somatophobia" in Western philosophy, a fear that the body is "a source of interference in, and a danger to, the operations of reason."[27] While this fear clearly predates the seventeenth century (going back at least to the primacy of form over matter in Plato), Grosz argues that Descartes intensifies this fear by not only separating mind from body but also separating mind from the very context and constraints of nature itself. This constitutes nothing less than a scientific revolution in which the concerns of the subject could be cleanly excised from the domain of reliable knowledge, where the knower could be "entirely . . . distinct" from her body.[28] Now, the mind can operate in isolation and purity, a purity unavailable to the unrealizable ideals of the Platonic form. From here, scientific (and philosophical) inquiry could aspire to a pure reason, and the failure of bodies to live up to this purity could attest to the superiority of mind over body, of ideas over practices, of "consciousness . . . above corporeality."[29]

Grosz argues that the result has been a reductionism—an attempt to explain the body in terms of mind, and to violently insist that the body live up to the ideals of purity and autonomy now driving scientific practice. In the liberal tradition, this amounts to seeing the body as an object—a tool, a machine, or a possession of a sovereign individual will.[30] And for Grosz, this reduction of the body becomes a fear of the body when the operations of the body visibly call into question the sovereignty of the mind. The functions of the body such as eating, sweating, and defecating, she argues, "attest to the permeability of the body" and thus "affront a subject's aspiration toward autonomy and self-identity."[31] Bodily secretions—the subject of Elias's manners—not only cross the increasingly policed border between self and world, but their viscosity also means they evade clear distinction and quantification; they escape the reificatory drive of capitalist ontology. They do not have fixed and stable borders and as such cannot be classified and quantified the way solids can. They escape the precise measurements increasingly prized in a bureaucratized and mechanized social order. They also betray the inescapable dependence of individual and collective life on the subjective and pathological domain of the material, as the secretion of fluids and the inevitable drive of hunger cannot—despite the pleas of rationalist liberalism—be overcome. The body, in other words, betrays two increasingly important narratives: first, that of a capitalist ontology predicated on precise measurement, and second, that of a liberal politics predicated on autonomous individuals.

Bordo and Grosz argue that this somatophobia is not merely misogyny (though it is also that). It is also a fear of the fragility of the narrative of possessive individualism that is increasingly being called on to order social and political life. The retreat from the body in both philosophical and social life, in other words, bolsters the emergent institutions of representative government and capitalist exchange. The epistemological concerns of Cartesian doubt, the political concerns over the measurement and demarcation of property, and the aesthetic concerns of propriety and manners are all of a piece; they all express the same concerns over the institutions of liberalism to ensure domestic tranquility and economic development. What appears as hygiene, in other words, is actually the ideological expression of the demands of bourgeois economics, or what we might, following William Connolly, call "liberal ontopolitics."[32]

The Work of Digestion

Though Bordo claims to capture the spirit of the modern age in Descartes's prioritization of mind over body, the social and political institutions of modern liberalism probably owe less to Descartes than to another seventeenth-century writer—John Locke. While Descartes provides a specifically epistemological defense of liberalism by linking the possibility of reliable knowledge to a theory of individual auton-omy, Locke emphasizes the specifically political dimension of liberal ontopolitics by linking a consonant model of the sovereign individual to arguments for private property, individual liberty, and representative government.

In chapter 27 of his *Essay Concerning Human Understanding*, Locke endeavors to explain what gives a person his or her identity—what dis-tinguishes one being from another and what distinguishes self from world.[33] He quickly admits that eating and other processes like excretion, growth, respiration, and injury pose an immediate problem for identity since they disrupt the most obvious ground for identity: the maintenance of the same body, or what he calls "identity of substance." Summarily, we cannot root identity in an occupation of the same body over time since, through these basic metabolic processes, the substantial makeup of our body is always changing. And yet identity—conclusive evidence that we are "that very same thing" from one day to the next—*must* be established, Locke argues, since political order depends on it: "In this *personal Identity* is founded all the Right and Justice of Reward and Pun-ishment."[34] Unlike Rawls's insistence that liberalism can (and should) be defended on political rather than metaphysical grounds,[35] Locke translates the political demands of liberalism into a metaphysical com-mitment to individualism.

Locke achieves this translation by arguing that we maintain a singu-lar identity not by maintaining a consistent body, but by maintaining a consistent "life." The "variation of great parcels of Matter alters not the Identity"[36] since identity is not reducible to bodily integrity; a living being remains self-identical insofar as it participates in a constant life. The "life" of a body does not change when it loses a limb, goes to the bathroom, or ingests protein, since these processes and their effects are subsumed under an organizing principle of the organism. Locke defends this claim at length through the example of a tree, which remains the same tree over time because it has

> such an Organization of those parts, as is fit to receive, and distribute
> nourishment, so as to continue, and frame the Wood, Bark, and Leaves,
> *etc.*, of an Oak, in which consists the vegetable Life. That being then one
> Plant which has such an Organization of Parts in one coherent Body, par-
> taking of one Common Life, it continues to be the same Plant, as long as
> it partakes of the same Life, though that Life be communicated to new

Particles of Matter vitally united to the living Plant, in a like continued Organization, conformable to that sort of Plants. For this Organization, being at any one instant in any one Collection of *Matter*, is in that particular concrete distinguished from all other, and is that individual Life . . . [I]t has that Identity.[37]

There are two salient points in this passage. First, and most obviously, it trades in the dualism identified by Bordo and Grosz, even while adhering to the pretense of an appreciation of the body. Locke is not entirely consistent on this point; sometimes he conveys a clear hierarchy of mind over body, while other times he invokes a third factor that seems reducible to neither.[38] Lacking a *principium individuationis* that is rooted in the body, Locke speaks instead about "Life," a vital force that is not contained within the body. But later in this chapter, Locke abandons the "identity of Life" standard for a more clearly rationalistic grounding—"identity of Consciousness"—and he glides from one declarative sentence to another, each more dismissive of the body than the last: "Identity of the same *Man* consists . . . in nothing but a participation of the same continued Life";[39] "consciousness . . . unites Existences, and Actions, very remote in time, into the same Person";[40] "*personal Identity* consists . . . not in the Identity of Substance, but . . . in the Identity of *consciousness*";[41] and finally, "it is impossible to make personal Identity to consist in anything but consciousness."[42]

Second, the passage makes a conspicuous shift from talking about animals to talking about plants. The reason(s) for this shift are unclear—everything he says about the absorption of nutrients (incorporation) by a tree could just as easily be said about a human (though the reverse is not true, since his thoughts on personal identity cannot hold for things that lack consciousness). Similarly, when he talks about loss (discorporation), he invariably talks about momentous extractions (such as amputation or hypnosis) rather than mundane excretions (such as defecation or forgetting). Though the subject of his study is individual persons, he shifts to talking about plants when it comes time to consider nutrition and digestion.

All of which is to say that Locke offers a very sterile and abstracted picture of continued life. Locke defuses the issue that bodies engage in material transactions with their environments as a matter of course, suggesting that these transactions are incidental or anomalous to the maintenance of "the same continued Life" rather than its very precondition.

He dismisses what Grosz points out—that living bodies steadfastly refuse to embody the categories of discrete identities—and he emerges with a sterilized picture of the individual being whose bleeding, suffering, forgetting, or growing is but a side effect of maintaining an individual, self-identical consciousness. Again, because "all the Right and Justice of Reward and Punishment" depends on clear, uncompromised barriers between the self and the world, and because these barriers are not available in the realm of the body, the body becomes a variation from (or a liability to) his liberalism.[43]

One might argue that this is mere discretion or prudishness on Locke's part; talking about digestion and excretion would have been inappropriate to a formal philosophical treatise in the seventeenth century (and may well be today). Maybe Locke is merely being polite ("civilized") in neglecting to talk about bile and feces, blood and guts—the bodily secretions that Grosz identifies as a source of fear in Western philosophy. But each of these substances was a significant sociopolitical issue when Locke was writing—the subject of all manner of public debates, legislations, and treatises. Elias covers some of these debates. But the body's foul substances became part of the daily conversation of the French and Brits in the early seventeenth century, such that rich vocabularies were developed to describe them in the years leading up to Locke.[44] This period saw the first laws regulating digestive waste—the first public sewer systems, and the first requirements that individuals maintain private bathrooms;[45] and since food contamination was one of the first recognized dangers of expanded capitalist markets and professionalized agriculture, Europeans by this time had spent three solid centuries consumed by fears about rancid meats and other dietary contaminants.[46] Nevertheless, even when his object of study is bodily integrity and individual safety, Locke shies away from discussing digestion, even though—and this is what makes the omission significant—the contaminating features of food were a great source of concern for his contemporaries.

Locke does freely discuss another way in which individuals materially transact with their environments: labor. In his *Second Treatise on Government*, individual actors engage in social and economic contracts legitimated by a presumption of sovereign will and consent.[47] But the political actions of these sovereign individuals are modeled on their laboring activities. Individuals domesticate the earth through labor, literally extending their bodies by mixing their labor with the earth and transforming the earth into their property—a prosthetic, legal, extended body. If digestion is the incorporation of the world into the self, labor is the extension of the self into the world. (As discussed in chapter 1, Bordo makes this same equation.) Here I quote Locke's familiar passage at length.

> The *labour* of [a man's] body, and the *work* of his hands, we may say, are properly his. Whatsoever then he removes out of the state that nature hath provided, and left it in, he hath mixed his *labour* with, and joined to it something that is his own [i.e., his body], and thereby makes it his *property*. It being by him removed from the common state nature hath placed it in, it hath by this *labour* something annexed to it, that excludes the common right of other men: for this *labour* being the unquestionable property of the labourer, no man but he can have a right to what that is once joined to, at least where there is enough, and as good, left in common for others.[48]

In the paragraphs immediately before and immediately after this one, Locke does talk explicitly about food: claiming that the "fruit, or venison, which nourishes the wild Indian . . . must be his, and so his, i.e. a part of him"[49] and stating that picking fruit (labor) and digesting fruit (eating) both amount to the same thing: a conversion of the world into part of the self: "He that is nourished by the acorns he picked up under an oak, or the apples he gathered from the trees in the wood, has certainly appropriated them to himself. No body can deny but the nourishment is his. I ask then, when did they begin to be his? when he digested? or when he eat? or when he boiled? or when he brought them home? or when he picked them up? and it is plain, if the first gathering made them not his, nothing else could."[50]

Shifting from eating to working, Locke negotiates these transactions between the self and the world through an intentional and extensive (rather than compulsory and intensive) activity. The shift thus allows him to subordinate the transaction to the presumption of possessive individualism—a presumption that both produces and legitimates an ideology of identity, authenticity, and responsibility that would go on to organize liberal thought and politics for centuries. That is, while one might read this transaction as a *loss of self* into the world, the politically necessary assumption of consistency of personhood mandates seeing this as an appropriation of world under the organizing principle of the self. As Bakhtin puts it, "man tastes the world, introduces it into his body, makes it part of himself"; whether labor is public and extensive such that self invades world or private and intensive such that world invades self, the result is the same: "The limits between man and the world are erased, to man's advantage."[51] In other words, whether eating or laboring, the process is the same: self mixes with world and world becomes self. *Self does not become world.*

Further, Locke's extension of the body by accumulating property facilitates Elias's measure of civilization: the larger your (proprietary) body, the easier to hide the metabolic tasks of labor. The acquisition of property—the extension of a prosthetic body—affords a very specific class privilege: the ability to conduct crude metabolic tasks beyond the view of any witnesses.[52] With such tasks relegated to a private sphere, the public sphere can hereafter be a space defined by legal contracts entered into by sovereign and abstracted selves, uninterrupted by those disgusting bodily exchanges that remind us of our animality.

Whereas Descartes posits the autonomous subject of liberalism by removing mind from body, Locke remains attentive to the body but negotiates a distinction between self and world by baldly presuming individual sovereignty and the subordination of the world to the self. One need nudge Elias only slightly to argue that the privatization of ingestion and excretion reflects an anxiety about the point at which liberal identity materially breaks down—where autonomy becomes dependence, where sovereignty becomes vulnerability, and where self becomes indistinguishable from world. Public eating and defecating threaten something much more profound than infection, disease, or lack of refinement: the ends of the digestive tract call into question the ontopolitical foundations of liberalism. In Locke, where individual sovereignty is the precondition (rather than the result) of the social contract, the threat of public defecation is not contamination, but a loss of the ideal of the sovereign self; not filth, but anarchy.

The Matter of Hobbes

But not everybody fears the body. In fact, though I have thus far used Descartes and Locke as foundations for modern politics, no discussion of seventeenth-century thought, of bodies politic, or of modern liberalism would be complete—or even credible—without Thomas Hobbes. Insofar as Hobbes stands as a harbinger of liberalism or a "proto-liberal," he presents something of an obstacle for a claim that liberal societies abandoned the (metaphysical) body politic for the (legalistic) social contract, for Hobbes was an avowed materialist who not only speaks frequently about the centrality of real bodies but also seems more willing to characterize political life through the idiom of bodies than contracts. As I will argue, this enduring commitment to a corporeal metaphorics (and metaphysics) explains the more ambivalent relationship that liberals have always had with Hobbes.[53]

Though Locke's ambivalent dualism and robust contractarianism all but completely abandon the metaphysical logic of a body politic, Hobbes relies on each of these competing metaphors; Hobbes would seem to occupy the very transition that Hale discusses from an organic to a legalistic worldview. *Leviathan* opens (and persists) by invoking the body politic, describing the body as a machine ("For what is the *Heart*, but a *Spring*; and the *Nerves*, but so many *Strings*; and the *Joynts*, but so many *Wheeles*") and the commonwealth as an "Artificiall Man" wherein "*Soveraignty* is an Artificiall *Soul*, as giving life and motion to the whole body; The *Magistrates* . . . [are] artificiall *Joynts*; *Reward* and *Punishment* . . . are the *Nerves*."[54] Hobbes discusses commerce as the "Nutrition" of the commonwealth, "the Matter of this Nutriment, consisting in Animals, Vegetals, and Minerals" that are imported and exported in line with the political body's needs.[55] This latter section is the most naturalistic use of the metaphor in Hobbes, as he discusses the imports and taxes as the "Bloud" and the public authorities ("Collectors, Receivers, and Treasurers") as the circulatory system of the body, thus charging the government ("the Heart") with the order and the very vitality of the nation.[56] But Hobbes's use of the metaphor is novel in a few respects. First, Hobbes is describing not an organic body, but a reasonable, prudent, and conventional one; the body is formed by individuals who *choose* to join it. This political order directly mirrors his description of the sovereign individual, in which competing appetites and aversions are negotiated and reconciled under the sovereign power of reason. At the level of the commonwealth, Hobbes describes a representational, rather than an organic, person: "For it is the *Unity* of Representer, not the *Unity* of the Represented, that maketh the Person *One*."[57] Second, unlike Platonic, Aristotelian, or Christian evocations of the body (politic), this body is anything but harmonious—it is a disordered, unruly, and contentious body always subject to disruption due to "the diversity of passions, in divers men."[58] Third, though agreement that holds the body together is between the various parts of the body (rather than between the individuals and the sovereign), the organs of the body are not dependent on one another so much as they are all dependent on the head (the sovereign). In sum, this body is constituted not by muscles, nerves, and common vitality, but by contract.[59]

This crucial distinction is easily lost in Hobbes, given his manifest dismissal of metaphor and commitment to the literal centrality of material bodies: "The World, (I mean not the earth onely, that denominates the lovers of it *Worldly Men*, but the *Universe*, that is, the whole masse of all things that are), is Corporeall, that is to say, Body; . . . that which is not Body, is no part of the Universe: And because the Universe is All, that which is no part of it, is *Nothing*; and consequently *no where*."[60] Historically, such materialism has proven problematic for liberals, for (as Frost points out) materialism, by disregarding the importance of such intangibles as mind or soul, undermines liberal ontopolitics and the ideology of individualism, threatening to evacuate agency and reduce to a crude determinism. But, Frost continues, this is only because materialist philosophy is typically read through an often-unstated commitment to Cartesian dualism. That is, materialism appears determinist if we think mind is separate from body. Hobbes scholars, Frost explains, commonly read a Cartesian mind-body split into Hobbes's account of the subject, even though Hobbes explicitly rejects this dualism offering not an inert or determined body divorced from mind, but instead a "thinking-body" that retains the ability to act.[61]

This rejection is visible in Hobbes's reflections in *De Corpore* on what gives a body its identity.[62] This chapter covers much the same ground as chapter 27 of Locke's *Essay Concerning Human Understanding*, though with a few notable distinctions. First, while Locke's chapter endeavors to explain what makes one person the same over time, Hobbes's text is more focused on explaining what makes two people different (i.e., no two bodies can occupy the same place at the same time; no single body can occupy two spaces at the same time); Locke is interested in what holds us together, Hobbes with what keeps us apart. This corresponds to their broader political commitments, as Lockean subjects are always threatening to retreat into private space, whereas Hobbesian subjects are always threatening to invade one another. Second, Hobbes refuses to root identity in any one principle (identity of substance, consistency of consciousness, or primacy of form). Instead, after rehearsing a series of challenges to both the form and the matter of beings over time, Hobbes claims that individuation is less an ontological characteristic of beings than it is a function of a complicated set of judgments about form, matter, and the totality of the being: "[T]he beginning of *individuation* is not always to be taken either from matter alone, or from form alone."[63] It is, in other words, ontopolitical.

As a result, Hobbes talks about this "thinking-body" being driven by endeavors and desires and appetites and aversions, some of which are internal and others of which arise from external stimuli.[64] Further, he is clear that when foreign objects enter the body (as in the case of respiration and ingestion and smell and taste), our bodies are "moved" but not altered.[65] When a second body comes to occupy the same space (as when a person eats an apple), the two bodies become one; one is subsumed under the identity of the other. Because Hobbes presumes the sovereignty of the thinking-body, eating, in the passing mentions he makes of it, clearly involves the subsumption of consumed object under the organizing identity of the thinking-body. Because he presumes individual sovereignty, *world becomes self; self does not become world.*[66]

This cuts to the heart of the long contentious relationship between Hobbes's method and his politics, between his metaphors of bodies and those of contract. Though Hobbes claims that everything that is can be explained as a characteristic of bodies, it has never been entirely clear how Hobbes gets from an absolute primacy of bodies to a protoliberal individualism. MacPherson famously argued that Hobbes's materialism and his individualism were mutually dependent; it is only by assuming the market principle of self-ownership that particular parcels of matter could appear as discrete and self-moving.[67] At the opposite end of the spectrum, Leo Strauss claimed that Hobbes's materialism and his politics were utterly unrelated to each other.[68] But as Frost points out, rather than reconcile Hobbes's "metaphysical materialism" and his "metaphysical individualism," most Hobbes scholars have simply presumed the primacy of his individualism over his materialism, focusing on "the Hobbesian subject *qua* rational actor."[69] As Frost tells it, interpretations of Hobbes are mediated by a concern that metaphysical materialism reduces all order to convention, and evacuates the possibilities of meaningful political agency. Hobbes became a "rational egoist" rather than a "metaphysical materialist" because the former is more compatible with existing political prejudices.[70]

I want to think Frost is right to claim that Hobbesian materialism does not pose a challenge to possibilities for agency as such, but it does threaten the individualist prejudices of liberal politics by emphasizing the unavoidable vulnerability of individuals and the fallacy of the presumed separation of self from world.[71] But this consequence of materialism seems as alien to Hobbes as is Cartesian dualism, a product in large part of the reworked understanding of matter and physics pursuant to the discovery of thermodynamics in the mid-nineteenth century in which matter and energy freely flowed into and out of bodies but was never created or destroyed. Indeed, Frost seems guilty of precisely the same mistake that she identifies in other Hobbesians: while they read Hobbes through the lens of Cartesian dualism, Frost reads him through the lens of nineteenth-century physics and its mobilization by Deleuze and his twentieth-century followers.[72] Her thesis steadfastly avoids the more familiar claims that Hobbes's version of materialism participates in the liberal project of separating man from nature and self from world,[73] that Hobbes continues to talk about identity as something that transcends embodiment,[74] or that Hobbes establishes as the primary political virtue the protection of individuals from violation and release of those individuals from unchosen obligation.[75]

Nevertheless, like Frost, I think Hobbes remains a contentious figure for liberals, not because of his absolutist political prescriptions but because his metaphysical materialism does not seem to bolster the ontopolitical presumption of sovereign individuality. And so Hobbes, read through the palliating Cartesian framework, becomes a theorist of the rational individual rather than a materialist. In other words, liberal appropriations of Hobbes ignore the fact that you are what you eat—or, more precisely, eating becomes a source of anxiety for Hobbesian liberals, and the inability of his materialism to provide a *principium individuationis* leads to a jettisoning (or at least neglect) of his materialism. Although Frost overstates her case in suggesting that Hobbes embraces vulnerability and creates a politics of intersubjective ethics, she effectively conveys how Hobbes's conflicted history with liberalism owes to his failure to be clear about the integrity of the individual.

Because Hobbes emphasizes how we are meaningfully subjected to material force, he adopts a political posture more defensive than Locke's; Locke seeks extension, while Hobbes frets about invasion. But Hobbes, no less than Locke, abandons the "grotesque" body in which the distinction between self and world is freely transgressed, and the digestive invasion that upsets individualism predictably makes scant appearance in his texts. For a materialist, Hobbes has shockingly little to say about what it means to metabolize and incorporate the external world; the one section of *De Corpore* that deals with eating focuses entirely on the physiology of taste and makes no mention of digestion.[76]

We might explain this omission with reference to Roberto Esposito, who stresses that Hobbes's entire project is predicated on establishing and protecting an ideal of discrete, bounded, and sovereign subjects immune to invasion from the outside world. Or we might turn to Elias, who argues that liberal civilization requires forwarding and defending an image of self-contained and corporeally distinct selves. In either case, liberal politics seek primarily to carve out and maintain private space in which to hide the ways in which we do not meet these requirements—a prescription exemplified by Hobbes's curiously sterile portrayal of the human body. So while Frost is surely correct to claim that Hobbes demands that we seek peace, her claim that he promotes this quest with an appeal to intersubjective ethics—an appreciation of our mutual constitution and vulnerability—is bizarre. Hobbes promotes this not by appreciating vulnerability but by aggressively masking it, by protecting and defending our bodily integrity.

Birth of a Metaphor

That the seventeenth century was filled with political and economic turmoil is familiar enough. As Strauss points out, this period marks "the fertile moment when the classical and theological tradition was already shaken, and a tradition of modern science not yet formed and established."[77] Phrased this way, this is (potentially) a period of excitement and wonder, where new scientific techniques and social power are afforded the opportunity to remake the world in line with new liberal beliefs, where sovereign individuals are afforded the power to create knowledge, value, and meaning. Said another way, however, this is a period in which traditional institutions providing social order are in decay, and new institutions that might supplement them are still being built. Said in yet another way, the body politic is dying, and the social contract is just being written. Not surprisingly, this is also a period of great anxiety, as the assurances of yesterday give way to the promises of tomorrow. In this context, as a new social order is coming to rest on the ideal of identical, authentic, and responsible subjects it might come as little surprise that demonstrations of individual vulnerability come to bear the weight of the fears of social and political disorder. Hence liberal societies were established primarily around the virtue of individual safety.[78]

In this new tradition—not only of modern science but also of liberal rights, of capitalist economics, of mechanical and bureaucratic standardization, and of bourgeois aesthetics—the distinction between self and world was called on to bear greater organizing weight than in the Middle Ages. This boundary was not any more or less porous than it used to be, but its porosity became less tolerable given this new burden. The defining texts of the era convey an anxiety about the bodily functions that compromised this boundary, and these functions were actively removed from the public sphere, and philosophical reflection turned away from the concerns of the body to a more pure and sterile realm of consciousness. Operations such as eating that remained invariably bodily were rewritten as private, more a shameful reminder of crude animality than a material experience of commonality. The individual that was welcomed in public was unburdened by specific corporeal demands and features, having sufficiently squelched those unruly and pathological instincts, processes, and secretions of the body. This was the abstract and sovereign being that could be treated anonymously and bureaucratically, could be responsible for its actions and beliefs, and could engage in regular and legitimate contracts.

This reading of seventeenth-century food anxieties draws considerably from the claims of Roland Barthes, Claude Lévi-Strauss, and Mary Douglas that food is not merely the source of bodily nourishment but is a system of communication that captures and reflects broader political and cultural dynamics about order and hierarchy.[79] It draws especially on Douglas's claim that concerns about dirt and disorder are more pronounced in times of political turmoil and that people express anxieties about bodily integrity when the boundaries of social order are themselves put under pressure.[80] The aim of this chapter is to read the presence or absence of digestive metaphors in political thought as signs of a particular way of theorizing the individual body that serves as a foundation for understanding broader discourses of science, politics, and aesthetics. "The mistake," Douglas argues, "is to treat bodily margins in isolation from all other margins."[81]

I am not the first to argue that the metaphor of a body politic is less consistent with the ontopolitical roots of liberalism, and so writers at the dawn of the liberal era traded this traditional metaphor for another—that of the social contract.[82] Nor is it new to claim that the philosophical ideal of individual sovereignty arose coterminous with the political ideal of national sovereignty.[83] But my argument here is that the texts that produce this ideal of the sovereign self and the ontopolitical foundations for liberal ideology do so by neglecting metabolic processes. These texts, coterminous with a series of norms and practices that systematically removed from public view so many metabolic transactions, establish a way of thinking about bodies as discrete and bounded that underwrites scientific, aesthetic, and political judgments about objectivity, purity, and privacy as well as the liberal trinity of identity, authenticity, and responsibility. In short, the privatization of food is but one instance of the retreat into private space that characterizes the development of modern liberalism.

It is telling that Hobbes, who has maintained a conflicted relationship with the history of liberalism since he appealed to individual rights to mount a defense of authoritarian rule, maintains a commitment to both of these metaphors in (seeming) equal measure. But his commitment is not equal; his use of the body metaphor is mediated by his commitment to the contract metaphor. Though he evokes a political body as a means to evoke a condition of political peace, his is a contractual body. As Flathman points out, the individuals on the oft-discussed frontispiece of *Leviathan* maintain their discrete borders separating them from one another.[84] They are not digested into a political body but are assembled and contracted into an artificial person. Comings and goings, transactions and exchanges, remain legal and discrete, rather than chemical, biological, or gustatory. As we will see, this contractual engagement offers a more modest vision for democratic life than would a more corporeal idiom.

Food in the United States today is, perhaps as much as any other artifact, invested with the rhetoric of individual responsibility. Coming chapters will explore how concerns about food today, like concerns about proper bodily comportment at the close of the Middle Ages, stem from an increased burden placed on fragile and quite porous borders between self and world. Indeed, I will argue that food anxieties reflect actual threats to social organization—threats to individual and national sovereignty—endemic to an era of globalization. But first, it will be helpful to explore how challenges to liberal ontopolitics have appealed to a digestive sensibility to break down the "invisible wall of affects" that stands between bodies. This "digestive turn" discussed in the next chapter will set the stage for a study of how eating remains an essentially public engagement, necessarily implicated in capitalist markets, ecological footprint, scientific progress, and the politics of international aid. If eating today is less implicated in public festivals and rituals of communion, trends in food politics have insisted that eating is a public act, and that despite the frequency of meals taken in the car, at the desk, or over the sink, nobody eats alone.

∃ THE DIGESTIVE TURN IN POLITICAL THOUGHT

WHILE THE SCIENTIFIC, POLITICAL, AND aesthetic discourses of the self developed in the seventeenth century rejected the organic vocabulary of a body politic for a sterile and hygienic model of social engagement organized around ideals of identity and authenticity, political thought turned positively bilious in the nineteenth century. Starting with Hegel's and Marx's concerns about alienation and coming to its apotheosis in Nietzsche's diagnosis of *ressentiment*, political thought of this period showed an increased willingness to call attention to the crude bodily functions that mediate the subject's encounter with the external world.

This turn prefigures the paradigm shift discussed in chapter 1, as a new understanding of bodies and force came to organize ways of thinking about economics, politics, aesthetics, and science. Drawing from the discovery of the laws of thermodynamics, the discourses of digestion in this period inaugurated a pecuniary economy of food but simultaneously threatened to undermine the liberal ideals of identity, authenticity, and responsibility. Whereas the liberal theorists of a previous era suggested that the most important organs for mediating our relation with nature were the eye and the mind, trends of the nineteenth century suggest that it is rather the stomach and the intestines—the sites of digestion, incorporation, and excretion—through which subjects make their most significant encounter with the external world. This turn offers a challenge to the ideal of sovereign selves standing above and reflecting on their circumstances, threatening therefore the epistemological demand for objectivity as well as the political demand for individual responsibility.

In this chapter, I argue that this turn to the gastrointestinal tract represents a paradigm shift that political theorists have been dealing with ever since. Like my readings of Hobbes and Locke in the previous chapter, here I read Hegel, Marx, and Nietzsche through the paradigm of digestion to show how their understanding of what it means to eat offers a specific model of subjectivity that reorients political understanding more generally. From this reading, the payoff of a book like Marx's *Capital* is less a critique of capitalism than a critique (as the book's subtitle, *A Critique of Political Economy*, indicates) of a particular way of understanding both subjectivity and value. Mining these texts for their digestive logic will help us understand, in subsequent chapters, how ideas about the meanings of self, space, and species are at the heart of both contemporary food debates and the anxieties of globalization.

The Digestive Turn

The shift from understanding society as an organic whole to a legal arrangement is arguably the most significant moment in political discourse of recent centuries. For though, as discussed in chapter 2, the term "body politic" has never disappeared from our language, it has, since the seventeenth century, been transformed from a metaphoric suggestion of the metaphysical unity of a populace (a unity quite at odds with the values of liberalism) to a rather more sterile legal arrangement mediated by the state.[1] The organizing political metaphor of modern society has undoubtedly been legalistic; even those remaining romantics, yearning for a period when children respected their elders or when citizens sacrificed for one another, consistently lament *not* the death of a body politic in which we were all essentially part of one another, but the cancellation of a social contract in which we all agreed to a rather more equitable distribution of risks and rewards.[2] Though contractarian politics have been subjected to critique since their founding, liberal ideology has grown so hegemonic that even opposition to liberal politics has tended to use liberal metaphors.

And yet revolutionary political writers have frequently found themselves in the throes of corporeal and specifically *digestive* discourses that more or less explicitly call into question the presumptions of individual autonomy and identity that ground the metaphor of a social contract. From Hegel's dialectics of identity and assimilation, to Marx's cast of economic exchange as a "social metabolism," to Nietzsche's diagnosis of bourgeois decadence as so much indigestion, one sees writers in the nineteenth century returning to digestive metaphors that upset the ontopolitical foundations of the social contract.

Much of this return to body politics owes to a renewed attention to scientific materialism between 1840 and 1860. Perhaps the most significant contribution here is Charles Darwin's rejection of mystical explanations for the origins and operations of life (both vitalism and creationism) in *The Origin of Species* in 1859. Though Darwinian evolution traces adaptation and mutation at the level of the species rather than the self, the theory still offers a materialistic challenge to the facile notion of identity that underwrites liberal ontopolitics. Rather than presenting a coherent self exercising sovereign agency in the world, as Hobbes and Locke do, Darwin firmly embeds subjects in a context, such that their existence is made possible by their dependence on and response to that world. In this paradigm, the self does not stand apart from the other, but is dialectically determined by it. Pollan illustrates this difference when he rejects the Promethean narrative of agricultural development as a triumph of human ingenuity for a characterization of agriculture as a "grand coevolutionary bargain" between humans and other species.[3] In this characterization, the spread of cornfields across North American landscapes owes as much to the ability of the crop to adapt to ecological and cultural opportunities as it does to human labor and power over nature; corn, that is, exploits people as much as people manipulate it. Medically, the influence of this evolutionary paradigm is most clear in the enterprise of immunology, predicated on the idea of *changing* the makeup of the body to render it more adapted to a potentially hostile environment. In other words, in a "post-Darwinian world," *pace* Locke, the self is neither identical nor authentic but is instead an adaptation to a given material milieu;[4] rather than "that very same thing" from one day to the next, "[t]he self is ever-changing as it engages the environment, exposed to potential immune challenges, some of which are rejected and others incorporated into an ever newly synthesized whole. From this processed dynamic, self becomes Self and is never a static, given whole."[5]

Less visibly, however, the period between 1840 and 1860 saw revolutionary changes in the study of human life, from the creation of the academic disciplines of biology and physiology (distinct from the more pragmatic disciplines of anatomy and medicine) to the discovery of the principles of energy conservation and entropy that are today known as the laws of thermodynamics.[6] The significance of thermodynamics would be difficult to overstate. The realization that motion, heat, light, electricity, and magnetism were all manifestations of a singular force (call it energy) quickly became the managing principle for both industrial progress and medical science. Kuhn has identified no fewer than twelve scientists working in all but complete ignorance of one another in the 1840s who publicly announced the basic principles of energy conservation—a classic example of "simultaneous discovery" and also a textbook "scientific revolution" that Kuhn would later become known for elaborating.[7] Kuhn argues that this revolution owes to three primary factors: the experimental discovery of the convertibility of magnetism, electricity, heat, light, and motion; the increasing dependence on industrial machinery for economic growth; and the popularity of German *Naturphilosophie*, which as a critique of Kantian and Cartesian dualisms sought to explain all natural phenomena with a singular unifying principle. In short course in this essay, Kuhn argues that scientific, industrial, and philosophical conditions were ripe for a widespread acceptance of a new metaphysics—one that challenged old dualisms, such as the supposed distinction between matter and energy, subject and object, and body and mind. In this new paradigm, terms like *matter* and *force*, which refer to discrete entities, dropped out of use among physicists to be replaced with fluid categories like *heat, motion,* or *energy.*[8]

Because his project is to explain the simultaneous discovery of the principles of energy conservation, Kuhn's study is relatively isolated. Though he certainly explains that this simultaneous discovery happened in dialogue with scientific technique, industrial development, and philosophical fashion, he stops short of placing this discovery in the relevant political context. Everett Mendelsohn, by contrast, notes how scientific treatises of this period demonstrated "a self-conscious concern with method, with philosophy of science which . . . is directly tied to a political crisis and to the movements and organizations which grew up in and around this [1848] political crisis."[9] In other words, this was an egalitarian science in which all bodies were composed of the same stuff, a science that resonated with the democratic rejection of authoritarian rule that was sweeping across Europe at the end of the 1840s.

These developments in physics also coincided with an unmistakable shift in medical discourses in Europe toward the digestive tract. Digestion proved to be the go-to variable for doctors in this period, with more and more maladies being seen as digestive in nature and, at one point, some 20 percent of all patients being diagnosed with a digestive disorder—diarrhea, cholera, typhoid, black vomit, or yellow fever.[10] Slightly more generally but completely in line with what Kuhn argues, nineteenth-century medicine was organized around the notion that bodily health depended on a balance between input and output—ingesta, excreta, and respiratory gases.[11] Hence biological studies of the period promised to relate specific vital processes (respiration, heat production, and muscle development) to particular ingested nutrients (carbohydrates, fat, protein, and oxygen). This belief in a bodily equilibrium manifests, for instance, in Justus von Liebig's influential claim that that muscular energy is the direct product of the ingestion and metabolism of protein, as well as Max Rubner's conclusive correction that animal heat derives not from a substance but from a measurable unit of energy called a calorie.[12] Whether emphasizing the conversion of matter (*Stoffwechsel*) or the conversion of energy (*Kraftwechsel*), both emphasize a stable equilibrium and reduce life to a singular variable: Liebig, matter (*Stoff*); Rubner, force (*Kraft*).[13]

As Rabinbach shows, this mechanical, digestive logic ultimately spread to medical, industrial, and political discourses such that each reduced essentially to strategies for manipulating bodies for productive efficiency. The discovery of thermodynamics and the standardization of industrial production inaugurated a tradition of dietary science and food faddism that remains today. As discussed in chapter 1, eating became characterized in an economic discourse, an activity quantifiable with attention to what is gained in ingestion and what is lost in respiration and excretion. This application of thermodynamics to diet was entirely consistent with the demands of a growing capitalist economy, both of which link success to the efficient use (conservation or transfer) of energy.

This paradigm shift does not *necessarily* violate the terms of liberal ontopolitics; a thermodynamic approach *could* justify hoarding *Stoff* or *Kraft* in a manner completely consistent with possessive individualism. But this would require seeing human activities as qualitatively distinct from other vital processes, a distinction that materialists from Darwin to Rubner explicitly challenged. As a critique of both the vitalist suggestion that energy resides essentially inside an organism and should be protected or enlarged (e.g., Hobbes) and also a more humanist sensibility that presents energy as raw, lifeless material to be acquired (e.g., Locke), the materialists presented energy as a protean animating force, such that even at its most acquisitive, the individual agent is vulnerable to, dependent on, and ultimately reducible to the forces of the material world. To the scientific materialists, we are not merely *in* the world; we are *of* it. In a more contemporary idiom, these scientists sought to "decenter" the subject such that is was the animating environment rather than the animated individual that was the focus of their analysis.

This application of this materialism to food can be traced to Jakob Moleschott's 1850 treatise *Die Physiologie der Nahrungsmittel (The Physiology of Food)* along with his own popularized version of same, *Die Lehre der Nahrungsmittel: Für das Volk (The Theory of Food: For the People)* published in the same year and translated into English, Dutch, French, Italian, Spanish, and Russian.[14] In these books, Moleschott explains food as the material stuff of existence, the raw building blocks of the body that are activated and converted into human tissue when mixed with oxygen in the blood. Vague or commonsensical as this might sound today with our knowledge of calories and amino acids, the scientific and political implications of this intervention would be difficult to overstate. For just as philosophical humanisms and constitutional movements were appealing to autonomous and coherent individuals exercising sovereignty over their own discrete bodies and wills, Moleschott reduced these humans to yet another expression of the matter that surrounds them. From here, human bodies are no more intrinsically valuable than any other sort of body as, indeed, human bodies are in constant flux, always transacting, piece by piece, with the bodies that surround them. Contra Locke, human bodies do not assimilate raw material in order to endure but are themselves only arbitrary compositions of primordial matter. In a sweeping rejection of the claims to identity and authenticity on which liberal politics rest, Moleschott summarily explains, "There is no activity without a constant metamorphosis of composition, without an eternal genesis and passing of forms. Therefore, I have been able to derive all life from the bonding and breaking up of the matter of our body. Life is an exchange of matter [*Stoffwechsel*]."[15]

For Locke, individuals maintain "the same continued life" *despite* this exchange of matter.[16] But Moleschott directly undermines this model of identity and, thus, the ontopolitical foundations for the social contract. Life here is not a function of individual bodies, individual will, or individual rationality, but rather emerges from a plenitude of matter that somewhat randomly gathers and disbands to constitute, reconstitute, and deconstitute bodies. We are not, in other words, discrete selves standing sovereign over our bodies; instead, we are merely specific organizations of the very same matter that surrounds us. Not coincidentally, Ludwig Feuerbach actually coined the phrase "You are what you eat" (more lyrical in the German *Der Mensch ist was er isst*) in a review of Moleschott's *Lehre*.[17] Much like Darwinism, this materialist reduction of humanity to mere matter continues to ruffle feathers to this day.[18]

This perspective would only be heightened in Moleschott's 1852 book *Der Kreislauf des Lebens (The Cycle of Life)*, in which he explains that plants convert carbon dioxide and water into proteins, which are then converted into living muscle tissue when consumed by animals—a process that ceases when individual animals lose the ability to replace their own cells. This statement of the "eternality of matter throughout the change of form"[19] amounts to a recognition of the inevitability and banality of death; as Gregory explains, "put this way, the life of the individual did not seem so very important."[20] Contemporary scholars of global warming as well as backyard composters can attest to the *scientific* merit of this position. But what is perhaps more important is its strictly *political* implications. Moleschott's realization suggests a commitment to egalitarian politics even more robust than that offered by John Locke or Martin Luther. For if political (proto)liberals offer a *moral* argument for democratic equality, Moleschott roots equality in the very fiber of our being. In fact, Moleschott provides a statement of *species being* that would eventually organize the thought of both Feuerbach and Marx: "It was a moral obligation to act first and foremost as a member of the species rather than as an individual."[21]

Moleschott thus challenges both the ontological and the political assumptions underlying the social contract tradition. First, the ontological claim to identity: the idea that we are a consistent, self-same being over time that can be held accountable for our promises and actions. And second, the political claim of individualism: the idea that there is some moral standing to pursuing self-interest. By focusing on the conversion process rather than the supposed coherence of individual bodies, he questions the very premise that our bodies are discrete entities separable from our environments. He challenges the premises not only of possessive individualism but also of individualism writ large.

Just three years after Moleschott's *Kreislauf*, Ludwig Büchner published what would become the bible of scientific materialism, *Kraft und Stoff (Force and Matter)*, which was translated into seventeen languages and reprinted almost annually for the next fifteen years.[22] Less immediately focused on the mechanics of digestion, Büchner's book proved a broad rallying cry for materialism over spiritualism, for empiricism over speculation, and for democracy over authoritarianism. Büchner's materialist account of bodies and vitality corresponds to Moleschott's concrete and demystified approach to bodies, casting humans less as functions of God's will or distinctive substance than as the transitory repository of protean and abundant material energy:

In the bread that we eat, in the air that we breathe, we draw in the matter that once built up the bodies of our forefathers; nay, we ourselves give every day a portion of the matter forming our bodies to the outside world and shortly after we re-take this substance or matter similarly given off by our neighbors. Of the English we can literally say that they gradually replay their forefathers who fell fighting for them and their freedom against the French Empire, by eating them as daily bread, for the bones from the battlefield of Waterloo were carted off in great quantities to England for manuring the fields, the yield of which was very much increased thereby.[23]

As a materialist, Büchner goes Moleschott one better, for if Moleschott reduces existence to a process of the exchange of matter (*Stoffwechsel*), Büchner explains it as an exchange of force (*Kraftwechsel*). Here, we are not merely moving and changing bodies but motion and change themselves. And while Büchner's work was quickly and widely denounced for its amorality and incitement to nihilism (if not so much for this puckish indictment of the British as cannibals), his more long-standing effect has been to unseat the ontopolitical foundations for a social contract predicated on identity and individuality.

As we shall see, these scientific, economic, and dietary discourses of the nineteenth century offered a dramatic shift from the discourses of the previous two centuries and exacerbated the political crisis at the heart of the revolutions of 1848. The stakes of this shift can be seen from an unlikely agreement between Locke and Nietzsche; for just as Locke admits that a belief in self-identical, discrete, and sovereign selves is required if we are going to allocate punishments and rewards, Nietzsche argues that the ideology of the social contract offers a route to social order by satisfying a desire to punish: believing in individual sovereignty allows us "to make [birds of prey] *accountable*" for what they do.[24] This new approach, by challenging this ideal of sovereignty, thus threatens not only our ability to punish wrongdoers but also the very idea of responsible agents that underlie established approaches to political representation and property rights. As we will see in the next section, as Hegel, Marx, and Nietzsche trace an ontology of static and reliable bodies for one grounded in the centrality of an ever-changing force (*Geist*, value, or will), they also call into question the most fundamental assumptions of the liberal political vocabulary.

Moleschott and Büchner, again, were not alone here. In addition to the dozen notable scientists, including Justus von Liebig and Hermann von Helmholtz, that Kuhn discusses as studying energy conservation, Darwin was offering a similar challenge to liberal assumptions with a model of evolution that reduced humanity to a mere mutation. If their arguments are distinct, and if the moral outrage has historically been more directed at Darwin, their broad ontopolitical implications are the same: to abandon the humanist presumption of an authentic self that acquires characteristics when it enters society. In a more contemporary vernacular, materialists rejected "the unencumbered self" or the "centered subject" of liberal political thought, a rejection that resonated far beyond the world of scientific texts.[25]

Though the nineteenth century is often seen as the century of the individual, it was the middle of this century that saw social dynamics and social organisms become an object of sustained scientific inquiry. After Auguste Comte coined the word *sociology* in 1830, sociologists would come to speak more often of a "social organism" than a "social contract."[26] Similarly, political texts of the day convey a more corporeal and organic sensibility (and vocabulary) than the abstract and transcendent selves found in social contract theory. If political thought of the seventeenth century was intent on explaining how discrete and autonomous individuals were bound to a collective only insofar as they consented, this period carried the specter of a preliberal organic whole, a political body predicated on the essential connections between people. If Hobbes and Locke root society in legality, political theorists of the nineteenth century returned to corporeality. In particular, Hegel, Marx, and Nietzsche each focus on the gastrointestinal tract as locus of the most intimate contact between the self and the world, as the point at which the external world fuses with the self and as the nucleus of ethical-political engagement. In these writers, political, ethical, and economic activity is best understood not as a legal encounter mediated through the bureaucratic apparatus of the state, but instead as a corporeal transaction of assimilation and excretion that mimics the human digestive tract. Value is not bought and sold, but appropriated and transformed; will is not traded and bartered, but lived and suffered; spirit is not managed and manipulated, but ingested and excreted. This is the digestive turn in political thought.

That liberalism's universal rights are extended to abstracted individuals artificially removed from the constituent environments and actual needs is a familiar enough critique, going back to (at least) Marx and up through (at least) communitarians and feminists.[27] And what I am arguing here is that the digestive turn marks a notable break from the abstract and bloodless approach to subjectivity found in Locke and Descartes.[28] By bringing attention not only to the body but also to the very point of the composition and decomposition of the body (the very points sheltered behind a shroud of manners in Elias's civilizing process), the digestive turn calls attention to the mythic premises of contract as well as the mystical characteristics of vitalism.

Locke does not deny these transactions, but they are largely irrelevant to his ideas about selves and identity. In Hegel, by contrast, they form the very constitution of the self. Indeed, while the Hegelian dialectic is often characterized through terms like *conquest, enslavement,* and *transcendence,* it is the metaphorics of digestion that structures and animates Hegel's project; his is a system of *digestive* rather than *possessive* or *sovereign* subjectivity.[29] In a passage on digestion in his *Philosophy of Nature* that directly parallels the organizational logic of his earlier *Phenomenology of Spirit,* Hegel posits that animals experience the external world "as *negation,*" and as "the feeling of *lack,*" and they instinctively attempt to overcome this lack by assimilating—*eating*—the objects they are confronted with.[30] In this process, the subject feels its dependence on the external world, and then attempts to overcome that dependence by conquering it, by reducing the negation to self. This conquest is ultimately hollow, however, since the negation that the subject experiences is not any discrete object that can be assimilated, but rather the finitude of the body and the external world itself. And so the triumph of assimilation is at the same time its failure; in asserting mastery over one's environment, one recognizes one's ultimate dependence on it. Attempts to maintain one's life require "the *immediate* fusion of the ingested material with animality"; individual identity requires "particularized infections" from the external world.[31]

This process of digestion mimics the dialectical *Aufhebung* that Hegel explains in the *Logic.*[32] *Aufhebung* consists of a cancellation, preservation, and sublation. In digestion, food is cancelled (as object), preserved (as energy), and sublated (as tissue). The point is not that Hegel spoke often about food (though he did), but that his project is thoroughly digestive in its *structure.* For Hegel, transformation is not the exception in human existence, but is instead the rule. More specifically a reaction to Kant than to Locke, Hegel nevertheless rejects the abstracted, disembodied individual bearing rights; and his dialectics does not merely acknowledge, but is predicated on, the failure of individual identity that Locke establishes as a sine qua non of justice. Locke offers a one-dimensional model of appropriation wherein humans acquire property by converting the external world to a piece of the self via labor. In Hegel, however, the external world is neither lifeless nor cleanly annexable. For Hegel, labor and eating are both processes of *Aufhebung* through which both the object *and the subject* are transformed. Whereas Locke endeavored to establish subjectivity (and thus liberal politics) *in spite of* the fact that individual bodies do not remain constant over time, Hegel establishes subjectivity *precisely because of* this exchange of matter in digestion. That is, whereas Lockean subjectivity is a function of autonomy, Hegelian subjectivity is a function of porosity; if Locke's subject is possessive, Hegel's is digestive.

This digestive structure is lost, however, behind the superficial casts of Hegel as a theorist of brute assimilation. From the beginning of the *Phenomenology*, Hegel warns against a perspective that starts with a subject and then ascribes characteristics to that subject; there is no subject without a predicate is how he puts it.[33] But when this dialectical structure is lost, Hegel quickly becomes the quintessential theorist of imperialism, as subjects go through the world assimilating all they encounter. Take, for instance, Alexandre Kojève's influential approach to Hegel: "The being that eats . . . creates and preserves its own reality by the overcoming of a reality other than its own, by the 'transformation' of an alien reality into its own reality, by the 'assimilation,' the 'internalization' of a 'foreign,' 'external' reality."[34]

While I think "the being that eats" is a good way to understand the Hegelian subject, it is telling that, for Kojève (like Locke) the fundamental human engagement with the world is not eating (internalizing), but rather working (externalizing). Though Kojève returns to digestive metaphors throughout his lectures on Hegel,[35] he ultimately downplays the way that the external world enters bodies (as food) and focuses almost entirely on the way that bodies enter the external world (through work). Though this parallel of working and eating is helpful, Kojève operates with the conceit that sovereign individuals intentionally and summarily conquer the objects they confront. In each case, the object of hunger/ work lacks self-consciousness and so is simply assimilated. Because of his preference for working over eating, Kojève is more interested in externalization of the subject than internalization of the world. And so in the end, Kojève's Hegel does bear the unmistakable marks of possessive individualism—the subject assimilates the world through digestion/work; otherness is overcome and reduced to sameness.[36]

Of course, Hegel's concern here is with alienation. The metaphorics of digestion, more than anything else, evoke a primitive reconciliation of spirit. When cast this way, the liberal fears of Hegel as an imperialist or preliberal authoritarian seem completely justified.[37] But as Tilottama Rajan points out, Hegel describes the complete reduction of otherness to sameness, that kind of total absorption and digestion, precisely as an illness: constipation.[38] Excretion is half of digestion; in particular, the half in which the individual reckons with the experience of digestion, accepts his dependence on the object, and "abandons the struggle" against the object: "Excrement has . . . no other significance than this, that the organism recognizing its error, gets rid of its entanglement with outside things" and expels the food and digestive secretions (especially bile) that are no longer necessary.[39] Digestion, not as an acquisition but rather an "entanglement" with the outside world, is the unavoidable condition of life and the ultimate demonstration of the dependence of the subject on the object. Hunger, as lack, may be a defect in the ideal of the sovereign self, but "the defect is in life itself."[40]

This defect is familiar from the now famous debates about the dialectic of master and slave in Hegel.[41] Similarly relying on the metaphorics of digestion, Patchen Markell notes the "tragic reversal" that follows an attempt to conquer the world through eating, "since consumption does not so much master objects as destroy them."[42] That is, though the subject may engage the world so as to assert its identity, in eating, the subject destroys the external object that would confirm its existence, leaving the subject "devoid of that external confirmation of its independence that it had sought. . . . For the consumer, satisfaction begets only renewed desire, and a renewed dependence upon objects of nature; and from this frustrating cycle, self-consciousness learns that it cannot find lasting satisfaction through the consumption of material objects."[43] This unsatisfying meal might inspire a never-ending drive to consumption and conquest (politically, imperialism). But Markell argues that such a drive could only arise from a simplistic misreading of Hegel's narrative. For Markell, the digestive logic does not suggest redoubling one's efforts to consume, but rather realizing that the struggle for mastery itself represents "a misrecognition of the basic conditions of human activity."[44]

Markell's point is that Hegel gets this—that the "very desire that animates the struggle for recognition is impossible to fulfill"—but it gets lost in so many interpretations of Hegel, in both criticisms and "stale" appropriations.[45] For instance, Alexandre Kojève, Charles Taylor, Will Kymlicka, and Francis Fukuyama all give a curiously triumphant tone to this encounter, arguing that Hegel promotes a "politics of recognition" that seeks an institutional setting that allows the manifestation and representation of authentic individuals. In the politics of recognition, justice requires that individuals be allowed to freely develop their own authentic identities and then to express them into political discourse and outcomes: "[T]he struggle for recognition can find only one satisfactory solution, and that is a regime of reciprocal recognition among equals."[46] This is curiously triumphal because it suggests that the resolution of the struggle between master and slave provides the institutional setting for justice; whereas, in Hegel, the section on masters and slaves leads directly to the chapter on stoicism, skepticism, and the unhappy conscious. (Similarly, the section on digestion in the *Philosophy of Nature* ends with a subject sated after a hearty meal but rather disgusted by its own feces.)

In Markell's reading, Hegel does not recommend the assertion and recognition of an authentic identity, but rather "a sort of abdication" of identity,[47] since the digestive logic itself is, to quote Elizabeth Grosz, an "affront [to] a subject's aspiration toward autonomy and self-identity."[48] The politics of recognition (like an imperialist politics, and like the liberal project of chapter 2) starts with "an aspiration to *sovereignty*,"[49] "the aspiration to be able to act independently, without experiencing life among others as a source of vulnerability, or as a site of possible alienation or self-loss."[50] But the digestive structure of Hegel's project is predicated on the permanence of alienation and self-loss. This is what Markell calls the "incoherence" of the politics of recognition: it starts with a recognition of the inevitability of our vulnerability, but then promises to overcome that vulnerability; it originates in a digestive and transformative understanding of the subject but then promotes recognition of our pure and authentic selves.

A politics more attentive to the digestive logic of Hegel, Markell argues, would be shorn of the sovereign conceit of liberal individualism, coming to a humble recognition that "the desire for sovereignty is impossible to fulfill."[51] The Hegelian schema therefore promises not an end to vulnerability, but a healthy appreciation of it. And for Markell, this digestive turn opens up to a politics organized around shared vulnerability rather than frustrated sovereignty—a condition of ethics rather than contract, of community rather than individuality, and one of democracy rather than constitutionalism.[52]

For its organic critique of the alienations endemic to industrial, bourgeois society, Hegel's digestive turn continues through critiques of liberalism throughout the nineteenth century. Marx relies heavily on digestive metaphors in his varied discussions of identity, labor, and commerce. This is sometimes polemical, as in the characterization of capital as a "vampire-like" parasite that "quenches [its] thirst" by "sucking living labour."[53] But more often, his descriptions of commerce as the "metabolism" (*Stoffwechsel*) of commodities[54] and labor as the "metabolism [*Stoffwechsel*] between [man] and nature"[55] suggest that the exchange of various forms of stored value—from plants to money—amount to the same sort of material transaction. John Bellamy Foster has done the most work on this imagery, characterizing Marx's approach to industrial society as defined by a "metabolic rift" that amounts, in more familiar Marxist terms, to the alienation of humans from the earth.[56]

As with Hegel, the logic of digestion structures Marx's very encounter with economics and economic thought; he explicitly reverts to its tropes in his critique of bourgeois political economy, and this theory of value draws directly from thermodynamics, holding that value is neither created nor destroyed, but is transferred from one substance to another via the activity of labor. Marx's appeal to "abstract labor power" in his economic writings follows on both the discovery of thermodynamics and the general industrialization of wage labor, as the qualitatively distinct forms of "labour" (*Arbeit*) are reduced to the quantitatively comparable variable of "labour-power" (*Arbeitskraft*); no longer a creative and unique human activity, labor in industrial capitalism becomes a mechanical transfer of energy (*Kraftwechsel*).[57]

Also, like Hegel, what is more important than his particular and numerous metaphors is Marx's regular reliance on the *logic* of digestion. In the notebooks he prepared for *Capital*, Marx identifies one of the blind spots in bourgeois political economy as the presumption of a clear life cycle of the commodity: born in the production process, distributed and exchanged in commerce, and then exhausted in being consumed.[58] In contrast to this model, Marx adopts a thoroughly thermodynamic model of the identity of each end of this process: "It is clear that in taking in food, for example, which is a form of consumption, the human being produces its own body. But this is also true of every kind of consumption . . . Production, then, is also immediately consumption, consumption is also immediately production."[59]

In many passages like this, Marx directs attention away from discrete commodities (which appear to come into and pass out of existence, as an apple appears on the tree and later disappears into my gut), and points instead to the quanta of energy that are transferred in each stage of the economic process. Marx cares less about the apple than about the stored and living "labour-power" (*Arbeitskraft*) that go in to producing commodities, the human energy produced by consuming commodities, and the surplus value than can be extracted from effective organization of these processes. Marx does not care about objects or the boundaries that ostensibly separate them; he cares about the energy that flows through them and the processes through which that energy can be metabolized.

This is no accident. Marx was intimately familiar with and interested in the works of Moleschott and Büchner.[60] Büchner's *Kraft und Stoff* was two years old and at the height of its popularity when Marx was preparing these notebooks, and one can see Marx appropriating Büchner's metaphors throughout them as he casts the human body as a thermodynamic machine, displacing energy in work and renewing itself through nutrition. Indeed, the ingestion and accumulation of food energy directly parallels the process through which Marx describes industrial production and capitalist exchange, as value is transferred from raw materials, machinery, and human labor power into finished and purchasable commodities.

This is, for Marx, a historical phenomenon. Under the condition of industrial manufacture, which is the specific focus of *Capital*, it is entirely appropriate to calculate *not* specific labors and laboring powers but rather "abstract labour-power," such that a bodily economy could be easily quantifiable and measurable and the bodily equilibrium sought by Liebig and Rubner could structure to the capitalist pursuit of profit: "In the course of this activity, i.e., labour, a definite quantity of human muscle, nerve, brain, etc. is expended, and these things have to be replaced. Since more is expended, more must be received. . . . [I]n a given country at a given period, the average amount of means of subsistence necessary for the worker is a known *datum*."[61] The consistent extraction of surplus depends on knowing this *datum*; a healthy economy, like a healthy body, depends on leveraging the equilibrium of inputs and outputs. This demand for consistent quantification also explains why, for Marx, understanding capitalism requires studying labor-power (*Arbeitskraft*) rather than labor (*Arbeit*)—the latter a series of qualitatively distinct activities, the former a quantifiable and exchangeable commodity measured in either hours or calories.[62]

In this model of *Stoffwechsel* or *Kraftwechsel*, production and exchange trade not in objects but in values, which are themselves "congealed labour-time."[63] Marx's labor theory of value appears entirely consistent with the laws of thermodynamics, where energy/value is neither created nor destroyed but merely transferred from one "bearer" (*träger*) to another.[64] Marx calculates the value of labor-power (*Arbeitskraft*) just like he does of any other commodity: it is equal to "the amount of objectified labour contained in [the worker's] vital forces";[65] "the value of labour-power is the value of the means of subsistence necessary for the maintenance of its owner."[66] Labor, like eating, is the metabolism of energy—that is, the transformation of value from one form to another; workers digest raw materials and excrete finished commodities. Whereas Marx's admittedly fragmented discussions of "productive consumption" and "consumptive production"[67] point to the metabolic equivalence of eating and working in part by noting how "production creates . . . the consumer,"[68] anxious works like Locke's and Kojève's characterize metabolism almost exclusively as an *externalization* of the self and neglect the *internalization* of the other. Locke and Kojève thus seem like artifacts of Foster's metabolic rift, wherein human beings, aided by the prosthetic advances of an industrial economy, imagine themselves to be decisively removed from the natural process of digestion.

Because it would invalidate so many political commitments to human emancipation, however, Marx seems at best ambivalent about describing human activity as no different from that of productive machinery and natural processes. Marx's consistency is shattered by a residual humanism in which human labor retains its creative potential as the source of new or "surplus" value.[69] He betrays no such ambivalence, however, in exploring how this approach to bodies and digestion informs a distinctly illiberal and properly communist politics. Marx historicizes this politics in chapter 13 of the first volume of *Capital* when he roots class consciousness in the experience of industrial manufacture when the discrete individual body is no longer the center of production. Because labor is no longer the creative expression of individual will but is instead a collaborative, mechanized, and standardized process, the material foundation for liberal ideology is growing obsolete. When people do not produce as individuals, they will cease to see themselves as individuals; the pristine, contractual subject of Lockean theory, appropriate to an age of yeoman farming, has no place here. Because what drives industrial production is not individual will or talent, but instead anonymous and protean energies that flow into and out of workers' bodies, the individual body ceases to appear as a discrete and autonomous substance. Marx's digestive turn suggests a homologous compromise of our individuality in the act of eating and the act of labor or economic exchange. In each case, the supposed identity of self breaks down, and what is revealed is our shared composition by impersonal material force.

This critique of liberal identity is further elaborated by Georg Lukács, who argues that the familiar model of objects as discrete and quantifiable is a function of the capitalist imperative for quantification and easy exchange.[70] The image of a fresh apple as a discrete object with specific and quantifiable properties rather than a storehouse of transferable energy, according to Lukács, owes less to the qualities of the apple than to an imperative of market economies to classify and measure objects for equal exchange. As discussed in chapter 2, Bordo calls this "objectification"; Lukács calls it "reification"; Marx calls it "fetishism."[71] The digestive turn rejects this move, casting economics, aesthetics, epistemology, and politics as a function of force rather than bodies, of time rather than space, of difference rather than identity, and of community rather than individualism. As in Hegel, this approach challenges the borders of the self that ground liberal ontopolitics, troubling not only liberal endorsements of contract and property but also more fundamental ideas about agency and responsibility.[72] Again, this is a digestive, rather than possessive, subject.

Marx's digestive turn might owe to his debts to Hegel and Büchner, but just as Kuhn noted a panoply of unrelated scientists simultaneously shifting their attention to energy conservation, Nietzsche's otherwise quite unique critique of liberalism similarly resorts to the logic of social metabolism. Nietzsche's penchant for discussing bodily fluids hardly needs to be rehearsed, but it is worth noting that these references are not limited to blood: he also talks about bile, digestion, indigestion, and nausea. "A strong and well-constituted man," Nietzsche characteristically declares, "digests his experiences (his deeds and misdeeds included) as he digests his meals."[73] While the extensive dietary advice he offers in *Ecce Homo* to those wishing to mimic his greatness seems at least somewhat ironic (given his well-known sickliness and inability to sell his books), Nietzsche frequently resorts to a rhetoric of digestion to emphasize that the internalization and incorporation of the external world is essential to the becoming and expression of human will. In *On the Genealogy of Morals*, he explicitly parallels learning ("inpsychation") to eating ("incorporation"), he compares a person who does not forget to "a dyspeptic—he cannot 'have done' with anything" (*wird mit Nichts "fertig"*), and memory as a form of willed constipation: "[A]n active *desire* not to rid oneself . . . of something desired once."[74] Indeed, reading Nietzsche, with his regular paralleling of intellectual and corporeal activities, one gets the impression that the malaise of modernity is but one big digestive disorder. Modern men, the *Genealogy* suggests, suffer from indigestion, anorexia, and/or constipation.

Whereas for Hegel that modern malaise was alienation and the digestive turn brought the subject back into communion with its environment, for Nietzsche that malaise is *ressentiment* and the digestive turn reorients the reader's approach to their own body. Nietzsche's critique of ascetic priests (as well as that of vegetarians and celibates) is precisely that they resent their own corporeality; they refuse to eat, believing that such crude processes contaminate their ideally pure body. Like Kellogg's pursuit of a frictionless and harmonious diet (see chapter 1), the priests ignore that "life operates *essentially*, that is in its basic functions, through injury, assault, exploitation, destruction and simply cannot be thought of at all without this character."[75] Whereas dyspeptics get sick due to an inability to process what they eat, priests avoid indigestion by pursuing a life of divine purity "floating above life rather than in repose."[76] Ascetics, in other words, pursue the liberal ideal of an authentic and identical self, uncontaminated by the ideological or material invasions of the outside world.

Nietzsche's critique of asceticism thus parallel's Marx's critiques of bourgeois economics, pursuing a pure and authentic individual self by retreating from the realm of material relations. Though Nietzsche does invoke "the sovereign individual" (emancipated from the imposition of law and morality and therefore able to make promises) as "the ripest fruit" of historical development,[77] this statement should not be confused with a liberal or Promethean ideal of a robust individual distancing himself from his context. The simplistic reification of this sovereign individual as somebody standing outside or above their experiences is only possible if we discard Nietzsche's broader claims that a healthy subject "digests his experiences,"[78] that one "becomes what one is" precisely through the experience of vulnerability,[79] and that one's mind or soul is but a conscious development used to put order on bodily experience: "[B]ody am I entirely, and nothing else; and soul is only a word for something about the body."[80] The liberal ideal of a self-reliant individual is "a fantasy of sovereignty" that animates the very *ressentiment* that Nietzsche is writing against.[81] In Hegel, the digestive turn is a response to Kantian idealism; in Marx, to commodity fetishism; in Nietzsche, to those who resent the very existence of their own bodies.

Like Marx, Nietzsche was quite familiar with the literature on thermodynamics (especially Moleschott and Büchner), though his early fondness for them and their critique of individual will eventually succumbed to a concern that their dismal science was insufficiently vital, essentially entropic, and ultimately disenchanting.[82] The conservation of energy, and the capitalist and industrial attempts to domesticate will, leads to an economy of decadence in which a frugality with one's own vitality leads to its decay. [83] As with the stale appropriations of Hegel promoting a misguided aspiration to sovereignty, one could draw from Nietzsche a reactive and resentful grasp at hoarding so as to stave off the vulnerability and mortality that is the inevitable condition of human life. But this, Nietzsche argues, is precisely why the priestly caste is so filled with hatred;[84] they are filled with an enduring resentment over the inevitable failure to live a life of ideality and purity.[85] Circulated in a world dominated by capitalist exchange and bourgeois morality, in which the aspiration to sovereignty serves as the bedrock of any notion of political freedom, a digestive philosophy like Hegel's or Nietzsche's might be seen as a threat as much as a liberation, rejecting as it does the very aspiration to (or fantasy of) sovereignty that has served as the sine qua non of modern political thought. In short, much like the overthrowing of religious political authority at the end of the Middle Ages, the digestive turn rejects the animating ideals of social order; if our very ideas of freedom are anchored in these ideals of identity, authenticity, and responsibility, the digestive turn quickly becomes nihilism.[86]

Nietzsche's response to this threat, however, is to abandon the conventional notion of liberal responsibility in which individuals are legally and contractually responsible for their actions for a heightened attention to the dependence of our selves on the moral and material conditions of our existence. It is this heightened attention to ethics that leads contemporary democratic theorists such as Melissa Orlie and

William Connolly to embrace Nietzsche in a manner similar to Markell's embrace of Hegel.[87] For Orlie, abandoning the "fantasy of sovereignty" affords new capacities for "ethical or aesthetic judgment" about the relation of humans to a vibrant yet vulnerable ecology.[88] For Connolly, the emphasis on the ubiquity of a protean and amorphous will serves as an incitement to generosity; recognition of the mutual and unavoidable vulnerability of human life is an essential step to recognizing the permanent and unavoidable condition of democratic pluralism.[89] By contrast, the assumption of sovereignty (Locke) or aspiration to sovereignty (Kojève) establishes a "transcendental narcissism": a pursuit of authenticity that ultimately justifies avoiding public life for a retreat into a sterile and contractually mediated private sphere.[90]

A National Eating Disorder

Hegel, Marx, and Nietzsche have each been recognized for their radical politics. What is less recognized is how each exchanged a set of ocular metaphors that have traditionally organized discourses of knowledge and self-reflection for a set of digestive metaphors that suggest a radical reorientation of the self to the world.[91] The idea that the world is grasped primarily through vision is consistent with the politics of representation, recognition, and detachment appropriate to a bureaucratic and, more immediately, capitalist order; attention to surfaces and borders legitimates an ideology of identity, authenticity, and responsibility. Digestive metaphors, by contrast, highlight the interpersonal vulnerability that is an unavoidable condition of existence. As such, the digestive turn marks a turn away from the conceits of objectivity and sovereignty; subjects are *not* removed from and looking at the world, but are rather implicated in and actually composed by the world. Digesting, rather than merely grasping or comprehending, experience, the digestive subject poses a direct affront to the fetish of objectivity in bourgeois science and also the possessive individualism of Lockean liberalism.

Martin Jay argues that what I am calling the digestive turn was largely German in nature. While Germans were working with the twin giants of Hegelian dialectics and thermodynamic materialism (ontologies of time and process rather than space and identity), French thinkers of the nineteenth and early twentieth centuries were compelled to come to terms with Cartesian dualism (an ontology of observation). As such, the French (with the curious exception of Henri-Louis Bergson) have tended to prefer ocular metaphors (metaphors that presume distance between subject from object, mind from body) to digestive ones. Note how when Kojève takes hold of Hegel, the dialectical engagement and struggle to the death becomes a narrative of representation and authentic recognition. Note how, later, Freud's narrative of identity formation focuses on the attachments and permeations of various bodily orifices, whereas Lacan's focuses on the exposure to a mirror.[92]

It might therefore come as no surprise that the digestive turn in German political thought mirrors the revolutionary politics and industrial development in Germany in and around 1848. The materialist critique of mysticism and vitalism in science and nutrition as well as the aesthetic turn toward digestive metaphors in political thought parallel both the breakdown of the German Confederation and the critique of authoritarian rule embodied in the revolutions of 1848. The establishment of republican rule in Germany, in other words, depends on a political critique of distinction that structurally parallels the metaphorics of the digestive turn. In his review of Moleschott's *Lehre* titled "*Die Naturwissenschaft und die Revolution*" ("The Natural Sciences and Revolution," the review in which he declares "You are what you eat"), Feuerbach claims that it is natural scientists—not political philosophers—that have always posed the real threat to authoritarian rule. That Moleschott, Büchner, and the rest were fiercely democratic in their politics is certainly no accident.[93]

Troubling the concept of sovereignty and all but rejecting the ideals of identity, authenticity, and choice that underlie it, Hegel, Marx, and Nietzsche all resist classification in the hegemonic terms of political discourse. Refusing to play by the rules of liberal ontopolitics, each finds himself categorized in terms outside of responsible politics: Hegel is an imperialist, Marx a determinist, and Nietzsche a nihilist. None, as their varied and familiar critics have it, contributes to the ongoing struggle for power and resources, nor even offers a coherent picture of human freedom. Insofar as political discourse is predicated on the ideal of the sovereign individual, it is difficult to render into political terms a rejection of this ideal.[94] The digestive turn, in other words, threatens the very terms we have for comprehending politics.

Beyond helping to categorize and situate these three thinkers, attention to this digestive subjectivity might also help explain why Americans today approach food with such fear. The pronounced unease that Americans feel about what they put in their bodies stands in stark contrast to the historical expressions of joy and celebration associated with eating.[95]

This is true not only among those suffering from eating disorders or advocates of those food authenticity movements decrying "processed," "packaged," or "fast" food since the 1960s, which seem a more or less direct response to the concerns about alienation found in Marx.[96] Nor is it restricted to the media panics over salmonella, *E. coli*, or mad cow disease. This anxiety has become a common refrain in the literature on the so-called French paradox, a term developed to capture the fact that the French, while eating a diet high in rich and fattening foods that Americans have been told to shun, experience comparatively lower rates of obesity and coronary heart disease.[97] The suggestion from this literature is that the French, perhaps due to a stronger commitment to social democracy and attendant appreciation for human vulnerability, feel the intrusion of the outside world as less of a challenge to their sense of self. The anxious approach to food in the United States seems grounded in a realization that the terms of the digestive turn violate the grounding myths of liberal ontopolitics and offers a strikingly different vision of collective life than social contract theory and the fetishized ideal of autonomous individuals. This is clear from the degree to which food anxieties today explicitly invoke these dominant ideals, as debates about obesity and diet appeal to an increasingly embattled notion of individual responsibility, exhortations to "buy local" herald the renewal of lived and governable space, and critiques of "McDonaldization" invoke a nostalgia for the nuclear family. Each movement reifies a liberal ideal; each refuses the terms of the digestive turn.

Of course, the digestive turn is not without its problems. In Hegel and Marx, it tends toward the sort of organic community that cannot help but be intolerant of difference; in Nietzsche, to the elitism that expresses overt hostility to the democratic sensibility and profanation of the scientific materialists. More generally, by questioning the grounding myths of identity and authenticity, the turn also throws into question the legitimacy of political discourses surrounding rights and representation—discourses, which continue to provide invaluable protections against physical and emotional violence. The turn, in other words, always threatens a return to a preliberal politics. We will return to these threats and the relevance of the digestive turn for democratic theory in the Conclusion. But for now, it is enough to note how the theorists of the digestive turn suggest an alternative vocabulary for conceptualizing another way of being in the world, one with an ambivalent relationship to real political affairs and the contemporary political imagination. Today, however, discourses of food draw implicitly on the digestive turn but tend more often to reinscribe the familiar terms of liberal ontopolitics—protecting and policing the fantasy of sovereignty where their predecessors rejected it. In coming chapters, I aim to unpack some of these debates to show both how the ideals of liberalism remain contested and contestable and also how the terms of the digestive turn might help us develop more adequate responses to the contemporary challenges of food politics.

4 RESPONSIBILITY AND DISEASE IN
OBESITY POLITICS

THE ANXIETIES PROVOKED BY THE digestive turn are far from restricted to readers of Hegel, Marx, and Nietzsche. When First Lady Michelle Obama launched a national campaign to fight childhood obesity in 2009, she tapped into widespread American anxieties not only about individual health and national security but also the degree to which individual habits and desires are manipulated by industrial food and marketing machines. Sander Gilman situates the current obesity debates in "a string of moral panics about food, the food chain, and disease which haunt our present age," as ubiquitous warnings about the dangers of sodium, *E. coli*, or high-fructose corn syrup herald our vulnerability to an opaque and powerful corporate food system.[1] Appealing to a supposed decline in individual responsibility, concerns about excessive corporate power and the spread of disease, the obesity debates today are rich with significance for understanding both the possibility and the actuality of human freedom under globalization.

In this chapter, I will unpack the terms of this particular panic and demonstrate how it is related to the concerns about sovereignty discussed in previous chapters. First, I situate obesity politics in the contentious debates about individual responsibility, arguing that the moral panic over national and childhood weight gain owes to a threatened narrative of individual sovereignty rather than a presumed public health crisis. Second, I explore the recent classification of obesity as a disease, showing how current food debates continue to exploit the anxieties of the digestive turn, even without reference to its nineteenth-century progenitors.

Ultimately, this chapter brings together the historical approach of chapter 1 and the metaphorical focus of chapters 2 and 3 to show how the arguments about obesity today respond to a series of broader anxieties about political life under globalization. The discourse of an obesity "epidemic," in particular, evokes salient concerns about the integrity of lived space, border security, and the reliability of the institutions charged with public health and safety. Obesity politics offers insight into—and fantastic resolution of—the crises of globalization, offering a biopolitical response to the breakdown of individual and national sovereignty.

The Meaning of Fat

In the spring of 2004, Morgan Spurlock scored a surprise box-office hit with *Super Size Me*, a video diary of his month-long experiment of eating nothing but fast food. Chronicling a deterioration in his physical and mental health that shocked both his viewers and his team of medical consultants, Spurlock's film became one of the top-grossing documentaries of all time, was nominated for an Academy Award for Best Documentary, and earned Spurlock favorable comparisons with Upton Sinclair when, soon after his film debuted at Cannes, McDonald's announced that it was discontinuing its line of Super Size products.[2] Spurlock's intervention was nothing if not well timed, coming on the heels of Schlosser's muckraking *Fast Food Nation*, a barrage of reports in the popular press about an "epidemic" of obesity, and the U.S. federal government's passage of the Personal Responsibility in Food Consumption Act of 2003 (a.k.a. "The Cheeseburger Bill") banning lawsuits against fast food outlets for making people fat.

Predictably, the film met with polarized reactions. While some celebrated the film's indictment of economic influence and the shameful quality of our national cuisine, critics indicted Spurlock for spinning a paranoid fantasy about corporate power and releasing individuals from taking responsibility for their own dietary choices. The film inspired vitriolic attacks and counternarratives from free market advocacy groups like the Center for Consumer Freedom[3] as well as from self-appointed hipster spokesperson (and, as of 2012, *The New York Times Magazine*'s Ethicist) Chuck Klosterman who, after calling the film "McDiculous," pronounced that "[t]he biggest problem with America is people who blame faceless corporate forces instead of accepting accountability for their own lives."[4] While one may have predicted such responses to a film dealing with such fraught issues as diet, responsibility, and consumer capitalism, the polarization took some peculiar turns. The most fundamental peculiarity must be that despite the frequent charge that the film releases individuals from taking responsibility for themselves, the film's final five minutes are dedicated to encouraging individuals to make wise consumer choices. Similarly, for a film ostensibly so sympathetic to the plight of the over-weight in "McWorld," its perverse voyeurism, with lingering shots of bloated thighs and stomachs, is clearly calculated to elicit feelings of ridicule and shame of the obese. But most broadly, it is curious that the film was widely discussed for its contribution to our nation's understanding of responsibility, even though the term "responsibility" (along with its derivatives and rough synonyms: "responsible," "accountable," "liable," etc.) is almost entirely absent from the film.[5]

In addition to being a hot-button political issue, obesity is today a guiding political metaphor. The meaning of fat, of course, has changed radically over the past century. I have already mentioned that the aesthetic concerns about obesity are, relatively speaking, quite new. In an earlier era, during times of actual or potential caloric scarcity, fatness functioned as a marker and symbol of wealth; from political cartoons depicting round men in top hats to resentful denunciations of greedy "fatcats," depictions of the overweight often signified an ability to sit idly and hoard precious resources. When, starting around the turn of the twentieth century and then especially after the exponential increases in agricultural production due to hybrid crops and industrial fertilizers, surplus calories became democratically affordable, corpulence ceased to be an indicator of class privilege and, as numerous scholars have noted, "fat became ugly when the poor became fat."[6] Today, when people are more likely to get sick from overeating than undereating,[7] obesity has become an affliction of the poor rather than the wealthy, and antifat sentiment certainly stems from presumptions about what physique accompanies such American virtues as self-restraint, hard work, and discipline. Yesterday's corpulent Mr. Moneybags stands in direct contrast with today's Homer Simpson, as the fat American seems today a ubiquitous signifier of both a self-satisfied, lazy, and decadent individualism as well as a bloated, smug, and ailing American empire. As Gard and Wright put it, "people have latched on to the idea of an 'obesity epidemic' because it conforms to a familiar story about Western decadence and decline. The 'obesity epidemic', so the argument goes, is the product of an 'effortless' Western lifestyle which has become progressively hostile toward physical activity and dietary restraint. . . . [This is] a familiar story which pre-dates by centuries the relatively recent spike in overweight and obesity statistics."[8]

But the health risks of obesity are also a relatively novel concern. Until the turn of the twentieth century, Western medicine was preoccupied with treating fatal infectious diseases like cholera and tuberculosis, and so studies of and treatments for such chronic and degenerative conditions as obesity, high-blood pressure, and cancer were still only on the horizon.[9] Even when diet and nutrition did capture the attention of the American medical establishment, the focal point for most of the twentieth century was not weight, but rather more immediately threatening variables like cholesterol.[10] It was not until the 1930s, when private insurance companies began to develop actuarial tables of life expectancy, that weight itself would be explicitly linked to concrete health concerns. The Metropolitan Life Insurance Company was the first to use a ratio of height, weight, and body type to calculate life insurance premiums, inaugurating the belief that extra body weight could have predictable costs and effects and providing an early articulation of what would become the now standard measure of body mass index (BMI).[11] This is also an early contribution to the neoliberal project, as the biopolitical drive to exercise control over mortality and public hygiene is displaced onto a private insurance industry instead of the state. The U.S. government did not begin emphasizing the health risks associated with being overweight until the late 1970s, and it has only been in the past ten to twenty years that weight itself became a cause for concern—not as an indicator or cause of other health problems like diabetes and heart disease, but a medical problem in and of itself.[12]

Obesity is much more than an aesthetic or medical issue in the United States, however. In recent years, fat has become an economic issue, linked to health care expenditures in the national economy and the adequacy of public accommodations for growing American bodies;[13] a political issue, owing to concerns about discrimination and legal recognition of the overweight;[14] a social issue, with the obese being blamed for everything from anti-American sentiment to global climate change;[15] and a national security issue, pursuant to an alarming report in 2010 claiming that 27 percent of young adults are so fat as to be "medically ineligible" for military service.[16] When Michelle Obama got involved, concerns about obesity immediately found themselves implicated with those other ill-defined cultural bogeymen: socialism, social engineering, and the intrusions of the nanny state. Indeed, in recent years, obesity has proven to be one of the more fascinating topics in American culture.

Given that Americans experience numerous threats to their health more significant than obesity and that the environment is endangered by forces much grander than a population's growing waistline, one could certainly see the fascination with obesity as a part of the ideology of diet discussed in chapter 1. As discussed there, this ideology of self-governance does not merely distract from more pressing concerns about individual control and self-determination, but actually shifts the terrain of politics from a public to a private sphere, where the operations of power are enacted on the very body of the participant. As neoliberal forces shunt more responsibility to individual consumers to ensure their own livelihood and safety, one might have expected a public outcry about a perceived cultural shift away from an ideology self-governance (supposedly signaled by rapid weight gain) or a willingness to relax the supposed border between the self and the world (presumably freeing people to eat more frequently, more freely, and less guiltily). In other words, and as Lebesco puts it, insofar as being overweight is seen as a violation of "traditional American values such as moral character, hard work, and self-discipline," the fat person is not merely a defective individual, but a bad citizen.[17]

The Politics of Fat

The story of how obesity came to be seen as implicated in everything from cultural decline to national security is a curious one. The statistics are by now familiar, repeated constantly in a steady stream of media alarms: according to the Centers for Disease Control (CDC), rates of obesity have more than doubled in the past generation, such that today some 60 percent of Americans are officially classified as overweight, while 30 percent are obese.[18] And explaining the origins of this trend has become a cottage industry. In one popular version of the story, propagated by figures such as New York University nutritionist Marion Nestle and Yale epidemiologist Kelly Brownell, the trend can be explained with such familiar concepts as corporate power and regulatory capture. Nestle and Brownell argue that legislators, regulators, health policy officials, and public school principals have become little more than puppets of "Big Food"—a cabal of companies that "produce, process, manufacture, sell, and serve foods, beverages, and dietary supplements" and that control "what crops get subsidized, which commodities get shipped to schools through the National School Lunch Program, what foods get emphasized in the food pyramid, and whether soft drinks are permitted in schools."[19]

Corporate decisions about the cultivation, subsidization, processing, marketing, and distribution of foods are all calculated to extract maximum profit, and because the number and size of companies that profit from the design and sale of junk food far exceed the number and size of those that benefit from the promotion of raw vegetables and modest portions, we exist in a "toxic food environment" in which Dr. Pepper and potato chips are cheaper than milk and fresh produce, and in which it is all but inevitable that large numbers of people will get sick.

A slightly more sophisticated but roughly consonant version comes from writers like Michael Pollan, Peter Stearns, Greg Critser, and Eric Schlosser, each of whom traces obesity rates to a series of social, political, and economic transformations since World War II—some of which, to be sure, can be traced to conscious manipulations by those standing to gain from the increased consumption of junk food but others of which cannot. Pollan and Critser, for instance, focus on how increases in agricultural subsidies in the 1970s were designed to lower the cost of domestic food and help the United States win the Cold War but ended up providing for a vast overproduction of particular commodity crops (especially corn) that would eventually change the economics of soft drinks and snack foods such that a half gallon of cola could become a typical lunchtime beverage. These writers point to technological issues (such as developments in seed technologies, which increased the overall agricultural yield and availability of surplus calories; the invention of high-fructose corn syrup; and the computerization of society, which created more sedentary lifestyles), social issues (such as greater tolerance for individual indulgence, declining rates of smoking, and the trendiness of baggy clothing that releases individuals from daily recognition that they may be gaining weight), and political-economic issues (such as large numbers of women in the workforce, forcing a greater reliance on packaged foods and declines in predictable family meals). This approach is particularly notable for its relative silence on issues of individual will or desire; here, appetite has almost no relevance to the issue of weight gain, which can be explained by economic, technological, and social developments independent of anybody's will. Indeed, individual will is even less a factor in these explanations than it is in the critique of Big Food, since in that critique at least corporate executives were conspiring against us.

These narratives about the supposed *causes* of obesity rarely if ever explore the *meaning* of obesity—that is, how people understand obesity, the codes through which obesity travels, or *why* people seem to care more about rising obesity rates than about many other threats to individual and public health (like the widespread unavailability of decent and affordable health care). Such concerns about signification have organized many studies of disease in general, such as Paula Treichler on AIDS and Susan Sontag on cancer and tuberculosis.[20] They have also animated a few studies of obesity, such as J. Eric Oliver's *Fat Politics* and Paul Campos's *The Obesity Myth*, both of which ask not why Americans are gaining weight, but what weight gain means to consumers, public health officials, and cultural critics. Of course, feminists have for decades been arguing that weight loss industries exploit an American obsession with slenderness for their own profit.[21] Similarly, Oliver and Campos both argue that the current fascination with obesity represents less of an actual existing medical crisis than an effective marketing campaign, noting how the overwhelming majority of weight loss products are consumed for purely cosmetic purposes, and how the American Obesity Association (which not only promotes awareness of obesity but also actively lobbies to ensure that diet aids are covered by Medicare and private health insurance) is made up largely of diet and pharmaceutical companies who stand to gain from a public panic over obesity.[22] Fundamentally, Oliver and Campos argue that there is no obesity problem in the United States— that weight gains in recent decades have actually been quite minor, that the evidence linking obesity to identifiable health problems is weak, and that the panic over obesity was manufactured by public health officials, cultural critics, and weight loss companies trying to drum up support for their services.[23]

While these stories certainly conflict in their assessments of whether obesity is a problem in the United States, they nevertheless agree that the current situation is a more or less direct expression of unchecked economic power. While Nestle and Brownell indict Big Food, Pollan points to "industrial capitalism" as a system that can "take its failings and turn them into exciting new business opportunities," and Critser focuses on the pharmaceuticals industry with his claim that diabetes is "the growth industry for an ever expanding nation."[24] Oliver traces the furor over weight to "the health-industrial complex" and Campos claims that the weight loss industry is "a fifty-billion-dollar-per-year con game" organized by "the dietary-pharmaceutical complex."[25] And this focus is ubiquitous: Ellen Ruppel Shell quotes specialists in "The Obesity Industry," describing obesity as "the trillion dollar disease"; Barry Glassner's study of our pathological relationship to food centers on the influence of "the food industry"; and Brian Wansink explains that we tend to overeat because "food companies" (including manufacturers, restaurants, and supermarkets) trick us into it.[26]

What these debates reveal, first, is that there is little agreement on the nature of the problem. Is it that we are too fat? Or that we think we are too fat? Or that we care too much about whether we are too fat? But a second issue to note is that upon scrutiny, despite their disagreements, it becomes clear that these arguments are linked by the shared concern about the relationship between individual freedom and economic power. In what comes, I will situate that concern in a broader set of anxieties about individual and national sovereignty under globalization. In short, I argue that what is at stake in these debates, and what gives them such purchase in the popular imagination, is the presumed threat to the assumptions of individual responsibility and representative government posed by rising obesity rates. The obesity crisis, in other words, is less a crisis of public health than a political crisis surrounding the viability of a Lockean notion of individual autonomy captured in the rhetoric of responsibility and the viability of traditional orderings of space and social order carried in the rhetoric of health.

The Responsibility of Fat

In the previous two chapters, I showed how philosophers as disparate as Locke and Nietzsche each explain the demand for a coherent narrative of individual sovereignty out of a desire to hold people responsible for their actions. In chapter 1, I discussed the ideology of diet as one particularly acute manifestation of this political commitment, as the idea that one could control one's body through diet betrays a deeply held conviction about self-governance and social order. Nowhere is this clearer than in contemporary treatments of obesity. That diet is subject to individual control remains one of the more deep-seated beliefs of Western society, visible in *ur-gourmand* Brillat-Savarin's claim from 1825 that obesity arises "almost always fall because of our own fault" up through Weight Watchers founder Jean Nidetch's claims that controlling one's weight is a way of being "in control" of oneself.[27] Blaming people for the shape of their bodies has a long and entrenched history, and the class blindness that allows diet gurus to claim that it is ultimately individual choice rather than economic pressures, cultural baggage, or geographic availability that determines diet and health is but one notable manifestation of a liberal humanism anchored in a belief that we ultimately own our desire and that individual health is ultimately a product of our own choices.

In such a context, it might be unsurprising the ease with which the obese are typically blamed for their condition, that obesity has become an unavoidable metaphor for moral weakness, or that the primary controversy surrounding the works discussed previously—most notably Spurlock's—is whether their explanations for obesity function as so many excuses for the failures of the overweight. Narratives of obesity rarely stray too far from explicit discussions of responsibility, and the narratives that seek to situate obesity in so many matrices of corporate deception, regulatory capture, postindustrial economics, or capitalist science are typically received as just the sort of exonerations that encourage a culture of irresponsibility and self-pity. Butler has addressed this dilemma of responsibility, specifically noting how the restrictive codes of liberal politics suture responsibility to individual causal blame, and ensure that attempts to *explain* situations will typically be heard as so many *exonerations* of the people involved—a dynamic that explains why Spurlock's film served as a referendum on responsibility, even though the film barely mentions it.[28]

Hence even as debates about obesity organically open into debates about public health and corporate malfeasance, and as citizens began exploring the possibility of holding fast-food outlets legally liable for the health risks of their products, the U.S. Congress intervened in 2003 to shut down this line of inquiry, passing the Personal Responsibility in Food Consumption Act, which proscribes any effort to hold food providers liable for poor health, enforcing the idea that obesity is an issue essentially reducible to individual responsibility. This unprecedented legislative act surely reflects a recognition that conventional narratives of responsibility have become tenuous—that formal action was needed to shore up traditional understandings of responsibility, to assert the relevance and adequacy of a commonsense approach to individual sovereignty in the face of a number of apparently quite credible challenges. This might also explain why, as Brownell notes, despite copious evidence supporting the thesis that obesity is primarily a function of environment rather than biology, public funding for obesity research goes overwhelmingly to biological rather than environmental studies.[29] Neither of these interventions promises the best diagnosis or treatment of obesity, but both promise to enforce a familiar, comforting, Lockean approach to responsibility that has been called into question by a widespread sense of economic and powerlessness in which people do not feel as though they are responsible for their own lives.

This suggests that the real stakes of the obesity debates in the United States lie less in individual or public health than they do in the viability of a conventional theory of individual responsibility. Looking at how the U.S. Congress and Spurlock's critics aggressively police the narrative of individual responsibility, it becomes clear that there are at least two reasons for this particular debate to bear so much significance for political life. First, the concerns about obesity are actually manifestations of deeper concerns about the maintenance of political order predicated on the ontopolitical assumption of individual sovereignty. This claim reflects the earlier discussed work of Mary Douglas and is further suggested by the frequency with which obese bodies are so often characterized in the language of filth and disgust. Lebesco draws directly from Douglas when she posits that obese bodies are figured as "dirty" because they are seen to violate the norms of a protestant work ethic, suggesting that the fascination with obesity today owes less to an actual or perceived public health crisis than to a concern about what appears to be a loss of self-control among Americans.[30] Obese bodies, which are presumed to be a product of gluttony, signify a failure to exercise the kind of self-control that is mandated by both Hobbes's and Locke's ideals of individual sovereignty. They also, by conveying a sense of unchecked appetite and offering a visible reminder of the practices of eating similar to burping in public, threaten the codes about propriety and bodily comportment found in the civilizing process of Elias. As Douglas further argues that enforcement of protocols that signify order tends to be most severe when social order is itself threatened, the moral panic over obesity and Klosterman's claim that it reflects "[t]he biggest problem with America" suggest a pronounced anxiety over the status of a cherished regulatory ideal.

But second, and just as importantly, the debate about obesity responds to the unwelcome intrusion into public discourse of that shameful and stubbornly illiberal aspect of human life: the body. The claims of the previous chapters about the prioritization of mind over body, the privatization of digestive activity, and about the abstracted nature of liberal political thought are borne out by the debates over obesity, as the shame and discomfort that often accompanies representations of obese bodies plays on norms of self-control and rational transcendence that the crude materiality of the obese body negates. Brillat-Savarin's classic reflection on his own "struggle" against his body remains true to the Cartesian dualism: "I have always looked on my paunch as a redoubtable enemy; I have conquered it and limited its outlines to the purely majestic; but in order to win the fight, I have fought hard indeed."[31] Confronted with an unwieldy, obese body that stands in contrast to the romantic, wasting, tuberculotic body described by Sontag as well as the controlled, disciplined, and productive body of Foucault, we are reminded of the unrealizable ideal of the sovereign self and the fallacy of the abstract subject that populates liberal theory. Further, insofar as obesity has been linked to poverty, being obese in public functions as a reminder of the increasingly desperate situation of the poor in global capitalism. The disdain for the fat is a disdain for bringing into public the reality and the unwieldiness of the body, for betraying the inequities of global capitalism, and for reminding everybody that their very livelihood is dependent on a corrupt and frightening food system.

One of the great curiosities of this trend lies in the fact that even among those most willing to explain America's expanding waistband with reference to geopolitically motivated agricultural subsidies and technologically rooted lifestyle changes, the narratives remain fixed on graphic and sensational descriptions of individual bodies and their grotesque habits. In *Super Size Me*, those bodies frequently function as moments of comic relief or collective shame, with lingering shots of overweight guts and thighs inexorably drawing attention away from the political economy of food and toward particular bodies. Campos points out that in books like Critser's, those bodies are often raced and classed in unsubtle ways, laying judgment on the individuals who fail to achieve the slender ideal of the abstract citizen.[32] Even from within the victim trope where obesity is just one function of overproduction and capitalist excess, the problem remains with *her* body or *his* diet. Even as Critser, for instance, focuses at length on technological and economic roots of the obesity epidemic, one of his primary arguments is that dietary literature of the past twenty years has shown a demonstrable trend away from the intuitive mantras about willpower and self-restraint—that the problem lies (at least in part) in a loss of an ideology of individual responsibility.[33] In other words, Critser explains why consumers have developed peculiar and pathological relationships to their food, but his narrative still ultimately indicts individuals for failing to control themselves, just as Spurlock still concludes that the problem is that people "choose" to go to McDonald's. Critser and Spurlock ultimately ask their audience to own their habits as they own their bodies, reverting to familiar codes of individual responsibility and thus reinforcing the ideal of self-governance to this political-economic situation.[34]

Even more striking in this regard is the literature from social movement variously known as "fat acceptance," "fat pride," or "size acceptance," which seeks an identity politics affirmation for the overweight.[35] The most visible contributor to this literature is Lebesco, whose *Revolting Bodies*, like Orbach's *Fat Is a Feminist Issue*, responds to the charges that being fat is a moral failure with the summary claim that it is often a conscious and empowering choice—an exercise in rather than a failure of individual sovereignty. Lebesco never quite delivers on the promise of her suggestive title (she never actually argues that growing fat is a *revolt* against patriarchal capitalism), but she rejects the idea that the obese body reflects a failure of individual will over material recalcitrance and maintains that being obese is often "the preferred way of being in the world."[36] Despite its reliance on the pioneering work of Schwartz (discussed in chapter 1 and thoroughly steeped in the language of orthodox Marxism), Lebesco and the fat acceptance movement writ large still pitch their claims in the liberal rhetorics of recognition, choice, and individual responsibility.[37]

In short, whether being celebrated or reviled, obesity today seems less like a biological condition than a metaphor for a biopolitical imperative to self-governance. In its typical condemnations, obesity signals a bloated and decadent imperial power as well as a lazy and degenerate individualism. But even the more critical treatments of obesity ultimately tend to resort to the same familiar codes of responsibility and blame, as they either flounder in their attempt to explain food politics without the language of consumer choice or reinscribe a traditional idea of individual responsibility through affirmative game of identity politics. Either way, the real stakes of the obesity debates are made all the more salient by their frequent references to the effects of economic power, calling attention to the threats to faithful representation in government and the integrity of sovereign states, while simultaneously revealing the myth of the autonomous self transcending its body. If obesity serves as a shameful reminder of the recalcitrant human body and its violation of liberal ideal of an abstract and rational subject, its biopolitical threat is not so much to public health as to the grounding narratives of liberal politics.

The Disease of Fat

Hillel Schwartz notes that the vocabulary of fat became increasingly vital through the twentieth century, as a notion of fat as a stable, inert substance sitting around the gut gave way to an idea of fat as a mobile threat attacking various organs, most notably the heart.[38] Schwartz sees in this transformation a narrative of declining control, as this hostile substance of the external world becomes ever more active and capillary, moving through and eventually contaminating the various areas of the human body. This vital notion of fat would come to its logical apotheosis at the beginning of the twentieth century, when popular, scientific, and policy discussions characterized obesity as an infectious disease: an "epidemic." Oliver notes the peculiarity of this classification, given that, at least according to standard medical definitions, obesity is neither infectious nor a disease.[39] But obesity is far from unique in this peculiar reclassification. In recent years, the rhetorics of contagion and disease have themselves come to colonize discussions of all manner of social and political phenomena, from computer glitches and the spread of information to crime rates and economic crises. The proliferation of this vocabulary speaks volumes about a changing understanding of bodies and space over the past decade.

The medicalization of obesity has taken place largely between 1999, when the *Journal of the American Medical Association* published a CDC study claiming that obesity is "a serious medical problem, increasing in prevalence, affecting millions," and the now ubiquitous claims that it is an "epidemic."[40] Exactly how many people's lives are affected by obesity has been a long-standing point of contention; the 1999 study claimed that obesity could be blamed for some 300,000 deaths annually in the United States, a number that was raised to 400,000 just a few years later.[41] These figures put obesity only marginally below (and primed to pass) smoking—the archetypal dangerous behavior—as a health risk. But the following year, the CDC's own Katherine Flegal criticized these numbers for statistical flaws and also invoked new medical treatments for cholesterol and heart disease to revise this number down to about 100,000, a figure that significantly troubles the thesis that obesity is a growing and mounting health crisis.[42]

But the specific diagnosis of obesity as an "epidemic," as Oliver shows, owes largely to the efforts of William Dietz who, while working at the CDC in the late 1990s, developed a PowerPoint presentation that introduced the now standard colored maps of the United States illustrating the rising rates of obesity between 1985 and 1999. With particular states colored light blue to indicate low rates of obesity, darker blues indicating slightly higher rates, and eventually dark reds indicating obesity rates over 20 percent, the slideshow depicted the United States (starting in the South) becoming darker and redder, with the dark and red section of the map gradually "spreading" outward across the entire country. This coloring has long been used by epidemiologists to represent infected (or "hot") zones, and this visual representation, still updated annually and available on the CDC website, "seemed to demonstrate that obesity was infecting the population with virus-like speed" and gave the visual impression that fat states were rubbing off on one another.[43]

Ever since, both professional and popular understandings of obesity have come to be colored by the rhetoric and logic of infectious disease. Indeed, obesity seems one of the issues to have been colonized by what has been called an "epidemiological imaginary"—a set of metaphors, images, and styles of reasoning that characterize all manner of social relations as so many contagious diseases.[44] In recent years, popular best sellers and business manifestos have deployed the terms of infectious disease to explain everything from literacy rates and sneaker sales to urban crime to global trade.[45] Of course, the rhetorics of disease and infection have long been implicated in discourses of communication and immigration, with the popular imagination tracing bird flu and SARS to Asia, mad cow disease to England and India, and AIDS, of course, to Africa.[46] But current articulations of the epidemiological imaginary appeal to concerns not only about national borders and global order but also to concerns about the changing nature of space more generally and the reliability of various physical borders. Invested as it is in remediating technologies of surveillance, mapping, quarantine, and containment, the persuasiveness of the epidemiological imaginary is surely related to the fact that the dominant political anxieties—from terrorism to immigration to outsourcing to surveillance—are focused precisely on the integrity of borders and the ordering of space.

Oliver's research shows how the discourse of an obesity epidemic trades in a fetishization of state borders and an assumption of interstate transmission, since obese populations are aggregated and calculated by their geographic location in specific states; it is the state borders, that is, that allows Dietz's PowerPoint presentation to illustrate a trend. But this convenient aggregation seems to have completely colored the way researchers and policymakers think about and represent obesity. Cutting edge research on obesity has turned its attention almost entirely to the transmission or "spread" of obesity. One popular strain of research traveling under the name "infectobesity" explores the role of viruses and intestinal microbes in causing obesity and promises to treat obesity with antibiotics or vaccinations.[47] Another, focusing less on infection but just as much on transmission, seeks to isolate the genetic preconditions for obesity, not surprisingly focusing on immigrant populations centered around the U.S.–Mexican border that are known to have uncommonly high rates of obesity.[48] But attempts to see obesity through the epidemiological imaginary came to their logical apotheosis in July 2007, when the *New England Journal of Medicine* published a study purporting to demonstrate "the induction and person-to-person spread of obesity"—not through microbial infection, but through social networks.[49] Explaining his work in the *New York Times*, principal investigator Nicholas Christakis posited that obesity "really is an epidemic," that it "spreads from person to person," and that his work focuses on "the importance of a spreading process, a kind of social contagion."[50] Obesity, in other words, really is an infectious disease.

Characterizations of obesity as a disease stand in notable contrast to earlier attempts to medicalize peoples' relations to food and weight. In a previous era, pathological relationships to food were characterized not in the rhetorics of disease and epidemic, but rather of psychological disorder.[51] Anorexia and bulimia, conditions suffered primarily by young women and widely attributed to either a pathological fascination with slenderness or a masochistic response to powerlessness, have largely been understood as psychological rather than biological problems. Hilde Bruch, the psychiatrist famous for her work on anorexia nervosa, similarly classified childhood obesity as a psychological disorder, largely a response to bad parenting.[52] Such a psychologization of obesity is completely alien to the dominant approaches to childhood obesity today, focused as they are on the relative availability of video games, corn syrup, and home-cooked meals. The willingness to medicalize obesity today reflects not only a readiness to see conditions that afflict primarily women as psychological in nature but also the mobilization of the crisis to reinforce the dominant themes of liberal ideology. Profiles of the obese today—even those moralistic profiles focusing on the quantity of soda drunk per day—rarely characterize their diets as an eating disorder, offering instead materialistic explanations about metabolism and caloric surplus, as if the fat body were a brute caloric machine, lacking any of the tragic psychic depth of the anorexic body. Today, bodies that call attention to themselves—especially bodies that call attention to the fact that they eat and, worse, eat apparently uncontrollably—are subject to tremendous resentment for their inability to live up to the terms of liberal ontopolitics in which our bodies are subject to our rational control.[53] Obesity makes public what is appropriately private: not only indulgence and the domestic (corporeal) economy and not only human frailty and the authority of desire but also the very activity of eating and the biological functions that reveals us at our most animal.

Such efforts to characterize obesity as a disease might sit uneasily alongside the cultural drive to hold individuals responsible for the state of their own lives, though it does offer the residual satisfaction of believing that obesity might be diagnosed, quarantined, and treated just like other infectious diseases. Nikolas Rose explicitly links such medicalization to a neoliberal discourse about surveillance, data collection, and policing public space, a claim that is validated by remembering that it was life insurance actuaries who were most responsible for developing the standard metric for determining a healthy weight (and thus the incentive to strive for it).[54] As well, with the privatization of responsibility for health care and the constant stream of novel weight loss supplements, drugs, and therapies, the medicalization of obesity further exacerbates the trend toward individual responsibility, with health insurance providers offering incentive to regulate diet and exercise and even threatening to decline coverage to those deemed dangerously overweight.[55] In this regard, the medicalization is entirely consistent with the cultural drive to individual responsibility.

The appeal and spread of this classification, however, seems rather independent of this cultural drive. Contagious theories of obesity exploit the growing concerns about the collapse of time and space endemic to globalization. In a discussion of postwar efforts by the World Health Organization and the CDC to track and contain disease, Kirsten Ostherr notes how the tools of epidemiology—data mining, public surveillance, and especially geographic mapping—not only represent the spread of disease but also provide intelligible narratives about transmission, risk, and political order.[56] By color coding infected and noninfected territories, such maps of disease reinforce an ideology of secure borders even as the story they tell is essentially one of their transgression. The CDC maps of obesity offer similarly reassuring (if misleading) representation about the spread of disease. In Dietz's maps, the condition appears to be concentrated in specific states, even though it would certainly be more accurate to show that it is concentrated in specific areas of each state and is better traceable by class rather than location. Further, in offering a visual representation of contagion, with one state's fat spilling into another, the discourse is easily annexable to contemporary concerns about globalization and immigration. Especially as the debate attaches to the raced and classed populations around southern parts of the United States (both the U.S. Southeast and the U.S.–Mexican border), such maps participate in a biopolitical discourse of race and citizenship, which is itself instrumental in legitimating the state power over life.[57] In other words, as the "hot zones" of obesity appear to be bleeding from one territory to the next, they simultaneously call attention to the fragility of state borders while also insisting on the natural and defensible nature of those borders.

In this, the medicalization of obesity not only attaches to established debates about individual responsibility and national security, but it also participates in a shifting political vocabulary. While totalitarian and preliberal societies have long relied on the metaphors of parasites and infections to characterize threats to the health of a body politic, this recent turn to epidemiology increasingly relies on the vocabulary of networks to characterize their transmission. The vocabulary of a "social network" invokes a kind of interlocking of subjects akin to that of the "body politic," but it suggests less that we are "dependent" on one another than that we are "interconnected." Stemming from the development of communication networks and the accelerated movements of both capital and bodies across the globe, the representation of a social network is readily implicated in concerns about the changing nature of space and, therefore, conventional ideas about sovereignty. This shifting vocabulary is also the case in contemporary social theory; from the opening pages of Jean-François Lyotard's *The Postmodern Condition* and through the more recent works of Bruno Latour and Hardt and Negri, in which social interaction is increasingly described through the metaphor of networks rather than contracts.[58] This shifting vocabulary might prove more significant for understanding obesity politics than revised dietary guidelines or intensified commitments to public surveillance. For as we shall see in coming chapters, the shift from a "social contract" to a "social network" as an organizing metaphor for political life has profound implications for understanding such issues as power, sovereignty, and responsibility.

Big Fat Lies

Located in a situation in which "so much about life in a global economy feels as though it has passed beyond the individual's control"[59] and in which "old standards of freedom and responsibility" are increasingly incapable of describing life in a complicated and often overwhelming network of power relations,[60] and with their multivalenced appeals to power, responsibility, and disease, the obesity debates seem less concerned with a public health crisis than with a breakdown in political order. Adapting Douglas, I argue that the fascination and disgust with obese bodies today directly reflect perceived breakdowns in the force of personal responsibility and reliability of expert and regulatory institutions. More broadly, the debates on obesity, rarely straying from concerns about a declining sense of individual responsibility and persistently deploying a rhetoric of disease that resonates with concerns about political space and border integrity, converge to highlight one of the more significant issues to contemporary representative politics (and representative politics more broadly): the question of trust. Interventions in obesity politics all more or less explicitly appeal to a wounded notion of trust among citizens increasingly cynical about the integrity of the institutions charged with ensuring public safety.

As discussed in chapter 1, the long-standing appeal of dietary literature to an American ideology of self-reliance has shifted in recent years. In each body of literature, from diet manuals like *Dr. Atkins' Diet Revolution* to political interventions like Marion Nestle's *Food Politics* to cultural criticism like Eric Oliver's *Fat Politics*, a common refrain is that neither the state nor the medical establishment can protect us from health complications stemming from poor diet. In each case, the institutions charged with regulating public health are ignorant, impotent, or (more commonly) irretrievably corrupt. The lack of faith in the established institutions of public health, now most commonly signaled with the dripping-with-contempt labels "politicians" and "the pharmaceutical companies," only intensifies the concerns about responsibility and vulnerability that are endemic to the debates about globalization.

Dietary literature has long traded in narratives of skepticism and quasi-religious awakening,[61] and the literature of the hormonal paradigm rehearsed in chapter 1 explicitly appeals to a lack of citizen trust. But texts promoting the hormonal approach to weight loss have intensified this concern; they do not merely repeat the familiar concerns that dietary advice is inconstant, but they straightforwardly indict the medical and scientific establishment for actually causing Americans to gain weight. Writers like Robert Atkins and now Gary Taubes recast the quite familiar indictment that official dietary advice is mistaken as a claim that it is actively pernicious. Taubes's *New York Times* essay that is widely credited with popularizing Atkins was provocatively titled "What If It's All Been a Big Fat Lie?" The double meaning of the term "fat" in this title is important, as Atkins and Taubes do not merely indict the USDA, American Heart Association, and American Medical Association for failing to stop the obesity crisis, they maintain that official dietary advice—especially the dogmatic claim that eating fat makes you fat—*has actually caused the crisis*.[62] Specifically, they claim that it is refined carbohydrates—rather than dietary fat—that causes weight gain, and that when "the establishment" vilified fat in the name of cutting calories, they gave rise to a national cuisine that replaced fat with carbohydrates. This carb-heavy cuisine, Taubes continues, promoted not only unchecked weight gain but most of the so-called diseases of civilization that are all but unheard of in preindustrial societies, including "diabetes, mellitus, cardiovascular disease, hypertension and stroke, various forms of cancer, cavities, periodontal disease, appendicitis, peptic ulcers, diverticulitis, gallstones, hemorrhoids, varicose veins, and constipation."[63]

Such a claim that the one consistent message from the federal government and the American medical establishment has actually been making you sick certainly appeals to an American spirit of rebellion, putting the Atkins "revolution" on par with bra burnings and the Boston Tea Party—a rebuke to the corporate behemoths comprising "Big Food" (Nestle, Brownell) and "the obesity industry" (Shell) as well as the state-market partnerships comprising "the health-industrial complex" (Oliver) and "the dietary-pharmaceutical complex" (Campos). Taubes, in other words, explicitly indicts each of the institutions charged with protecting individual and public health, and his work appeals directly to a presumed sense of powerlessness among American dieters, promising a measure of individual power through good old fashioned self-reliance and institutional skepticism. Again, he is far from alone in this approach: Nestle and Schlosser, figures as likely as any to discuss the welfare state as a protector of individual freedoms, identify so much corruption in the formal institutions of representative government that they cannot but place the responsibility on individual consumers to make wise decisions. Typically, the payoff of such dietary literature is a quasi-libertarian charge that the only reliable guide to good food is a local, autonomous, and uncertified farmer,[64] your grandparents,[65] or your own idiosyncratic taste buds.[66] Calling attention to the reliability of scientific expertise and public health and regulatory institutions, charging the state with actually spreading disease rather than curtailing it, this otherwise anticorporate literature has tremendous resonance with a politics of personal responsibility and decline in faith of the institutions charged with governance and public health.

These indictments of the traditional institutions of governance are of a piece with the critical literature on globalization and the decline in national sovereignty. Just as the sovereign, choosing individual is predicated on an ontopolitical assumption about a discrete and bounded self subordinate to a coherent reason, the idea of national sovereignty is increasingly called into question by the porosity of national borders, the subordination of state policy to the dictates of international finance organizations like the International Monetary Fund, and the purported wholesale corruption of the federal government by paid lobbyists and corporate lawyers. In this sense, the crisis of individual responsibility reportedly signaled by the obesity epidemic runs directly parallel to the decline of state sovereignty on display in debates about globalization. Maps of the spread of obesity reassert the significance of territorial borders and lived space, while public shaming of the overweight enacts the biopolitical imperative to self-governance and responsible consumption that, according to Foucault, was necessary as a supplement to the limited, liberal state.[67] In this sense, the truth of Klosterman's critique of Spurlock is not that Spurlock gives us license to be fat, but that he captures the primary dilemma facing democratic politics today: he calls attention to the failures of biopolitical order right as the sovereign state is breaking down; he troubles the grounding logic of individual and national sovereignty, but fails to provide a viable alternative (except a crude and inconsistent appeal to responsible consumerism). This explains why Spurlock seems both sympathetic to and mocking of fat people: he falls back on the selfsame notion of consumer sovereignty, even though his entire narrative rejects that assumption.

Most broadly, however, the characterizations of obesity as a disease, like other appeals to the epidemiological imaginary, reflect a shifting political vocabulary from that of a social contract to that of a social network. This shift corresponds to a breakdown in the traditional institutions that legitimate the contract—specifically, a belief in sovereign individuality and the integrity of territorially distinct states. But while the shift from the days of a body politic to that of a social contract required a corresponding shift in political logic—from one based in authority, hierarchy, and mutual dependence to one of equality, legality, and tolerance—the metaphor of a social network carries no obvious or explicit political connotations. While contracts, presuming both the sovereignty and the rough equality of all participants, convey an ontopolitical foundation for democracy, a network, presuming anarchic organization and level distribution of power, seems completely inadequate to capture the actual operations of power and politics in a global capitalist society. As a result, while so much of political life comes to be characterized as a network, this characterization provides scant if any resources for actually locating oneself in a matrix of power or an organization of politics.

Fredric Jameson talks of political vocabularies providing "cognitive maps," which allow subjects to understand their place in a political structure.[68] One way to frame the current controversy is as another articulation of the long-standing question about the politics of postmodernism. For just as writers like Michel Foucault and Judith Butler were indicted a decade ago for failing to speak a language of agentic subjects capable of expressing authentic interests in the field of representative politics, the charge now is that the vocabulary of networks provides no reliable cognitive map. As food discourses, such as that of an obesity epidemic, find themselves incorporated into this new, disorienting vocabulary, they increasingly provoke anxieties not just about how we eat, but about how a democracy can (or could) function. As much recent political theory suggests, though political life since the seventeenth century has been organized under the banner of sovereignty, the very concept of sovereignty seems inconsistent with the metaphor of a headless social network. In this context, the medicalization of disease signals not so much a threat to public health, but the emergence of a new political logic as yet incapable of explaining the operations of power or democracy.

5 THE YEAR OF EATING POLITICALLY

Wendell Berry famously declared that "eating is an agricultural act,"[1] and recent trends in food activism have announced that eating is a political, economic, environmental, aesthetic, and ethical act as well. While the obesity debates enact demands for individual responsibility and public health and so stand out as a marker of the cultural politics of blame, approaches to the political economy of food in the United States call attention to the ownership of seed technology and farm subsidies but find their popular support almost entirely around the demand to buy responsibly grown foods. Just as moral and aesthetic judgments about overweight bodies shifted over the twentieth century relative to new technologies of production and accumulation, a shift in the terms of responsible food at the opening of the twenty-first century—in particular, a shift from valorizing "organic" to "local"—reflects a changing nature of capital accumulation under globalization. Further, just as Hegel, Marx, and Nietzsche used a series of digestive metaphors to disrupt the assumptions underwriting liberal politics, the specific terms of food activism today reflect a particular understanding of the shape of the political subject and the terms of political engagement.

Current trends in food politics—in particular, the valorization of farmers' markets and the emergence of "local" as the badge of responsible food—often stand in uneasy alliance with the terms of liberal ontopolitics. In one sense, advocating an ethical relationship with the land and direct, face-to-face encounters between producers and consumers, the movement seems to promote what Murray Bookchin has called a "moral economy" in which decisions about production and consumption are guided by ethical regard rather than profitability.[2] But at the same time, exhortations to "buy local" correspond to a model of citizenship that impoverishes traditional modes of political action and democratic control. Reducing politics to consumerism and economics to ethics, current approaches to responsible foods and food activism tend to reflect the actual foreclosure of political possibility. By relocating political action to the actual and metaphorical space of the market, these trends reflect a subordination of political discourse to the terms of global capitalism and a neoliberal condition in which it is only in the rhetoric of consumer choice that Americans can imagine wielding power. These trends thus veer toward postpolitical fantasies that differ in content but not in form from the neoliberal promise of a harmonious society governed only by voluntary contracts and individual responsibility. Though food activism is typically couched in promises of democracy and equality, it often erects barriers to these ideals by charging the market with the responsibility for realizing them.

Despite the manifest overlap between the calls for "organic" and "local" foods, these movements are rooted in distinct idioms that respond to very specific historical conditions; both are animated by anxieties about the health of individual bodies and bodies politic, but the turn to locals reflects a realization that this health is threatened less by industrial pollution and nuclear annihilation than by the erosion of national sovereignty, the changing nature of political space, and the looming exhaustion of the earth's oil supplies. But like its predecessor, the dominant articulations of the promise of local foods reflect more than anything else a deep suspicion of conventional politics and the wholesale colonization of the political imaginary by the logic of the market.

Local Is the New Organic

Histories of organic foods in the United States invariably point to the 1960s, a periodization that owes to scientific, political, and ideological developments of the decade. Before the invention and rapid appropriation of chemical pesticides and fertilizers by American farmers in the 1940s, all foods were what would today pass for "organic." And between Rachel Carson's *Silent Spring* (1962), which catalyzed concerns about chemical pesticides such as DDT, and Frances Moore Lappé's *Diet for a Small Planet* (1971), which tied global hunger to the industrialization of the American diet, Americans saw a rapid proliferation of books and organizations promoting a return to small-scale, organic agriculture, and alternative diets (vegetarianism, macrobiotics) linking food choices not only to concerns about public health and global inequality but also to individual authenticity, social solidarity, and the ethics of capitalist exchange. Symbolized by the Robin Hood Commission's 1969 christening of a vacant Berkeley lot "People's Park" in order to grow and distribute free meals, the organic foods movement has always been firmly rooted in and hardly distinguishable from the politics and ideals of the 1960s counterculture.

If rooting organic foods in this romanticized decade is both convenient and stereotypical, it is also illuminating for its demonstration of how even this most idealistic of countercultures remained enamored of a populist do-it-yourself ethos and belief in American entrepreneurialism that has always evoked a suspicion of institutional politics. The liberal ideal of the sovereign individual, in other words, has marked even many oppositional discourses in American politics. Julie Guthman demonstrates this paradox in a comprehensive study of organic farming in California.[3] Guthman identifies four broad concerns animating the organics movement: the alienating nature of industrial production, the health effects of processed foods, the social justice concerns endemic to the counterculture, and the environmental impact of industrial pollutants. But these concerns have rarely added up to a coherent political program, she continues, and so while the movement has always been organized around a broadly conceived back-to-the-land ethos that was a reaction to postwar suburbanization, the movement has typically found itself promoting rival (and often bluntly incompatible) value systems—one promoting social solidarity and civic engagement, and another promoting individual autonomy and "agrarian populism."

Similarly, though Samuel Fromartz's summary claim that "organic food was supposed to be pure, wholesome, natural, and small-scale, a true alternative to conventional food" seems straightforward enough, it is curious that purity would be one of the organizing themes of the organics movement given that the foods the movement defines itself against—the processed foods and chain restaurants developed through the 1950s—were themselves promoted primarily for their hygienic and sterilized packaging.[4] Organic food and fast food both capitalized on an American "obsession with food and filth"; just as restaurant franchises promised the same hygienic facilities at every location, organics allowed eaters to "purge oneself of the dirty things modern eating put in one's system" by eating "whole foods" uncontaminated by artificial sweeteners, preservatives, pesticides, and hormones, and by developing a food chain (and eventually a national economy) uncorrupted by fossil fuels and capitalist science.[5] This attempt to heal Marx's metabolic rift promised a relationship with the land and one's food that was not mediated by industrial machinery, chemical toxins, or dubious profit-maximizing enterprises. At the same time, it traded in the ideal of individual authenticity endemic to the liberal political vocabulary.

Following Mary Douglas, we might read this midcentury obsession with dirt as indicative of broader concerns about political order. For not only did chain restaurants offer a cleanliness that fantastically conjured social order, but they also offered almost without fail the kind of meat-and-potatoes familiarity that reinforced an ideal of an American lifestyle in the face of disruptions to both global order and national culture.[6] Similarly, the appeal of organics lies beyond concerns about toxins in the industrial food supply, capturing instead much broader concern about the corruption of the natural and political worlds. In his history of "the countercuisine," Warren Belasco explains how the movement saw the corrupted products of the industrial food supply as symbols of the corruption of American society: "Wonder Bread . . . aptly symbolized the white flight of the 1950s and 1960s. To make clean bread, . . . bakers removed all colored ingredients (segregation), bleached the remaining flour (suburban school socialization), and then, to prevent discoloring decay, added strong preservatives and stabilizers (law enforcement)."[7] It certainly did not hurt that the same corporations targeted for producing chemically laden food (e.g., Dow) were also implicated in manufacturing the napalm and Agent Orange that were being used in Vietnam.[8]

Just like the counterculture of which it was a part, the organics movement eventually found its way into a more conventional capitalist market. This actually happened quite rapidly in 1989, after *60 Minutes* aired a report about Alar, a pesticide and probable human carcinogen then in wide use on apple crops. Within a year of this broadcast, the U.S. Environmental Protection Agency banned Alar, *Newsweek*'s cover declared "A Panic for Organic," and the U.S. government passed the Organic Foods Production Act (OFPA), establishing the first formal regulations for the production, certification, and marketing of organic foods.[9] Within fifteen years, organics would metastasize into a $15-billion industry with firms like Heinz, General Mills, and ConAgra owning some of the most recognizable organic brands and with critics positioning "Big Organic" as an industry on the order of "Big Oil," "Big Food," and "Big Pharma."[10]

One could certainly predict conflict and growing pains in an organics movement linked into both the 1960s counterculture and Reagan-era concerns about individual health. The linkage of organic foods and the struggle of nonwhite peoples might contrast dramatically with their contemporary position in upscale groceries like Whole Foods. But it was surely only a matter of time before Big Food found a way to capitalize on the anxiety over industrial filth. As organics grew, it continued to thrive on a perceived deliverance from toxicity. In either case, it promised reconciliation with a purer, more natural order that was threatened or abandoned by industrial society and the new technologies symbolized by Twinkies, TV dinners, and white bread. So like the 1960s itself, the story of organics is by now a well-rehearsed narrative of dashed hopes, capitalist co-optation, and corporate corruption, such that by 2006 retail leviathan Wal-Mart was selling organic produce and organic spinach had been tainted by *E. coli* 0157, a toxic bacteria that owes its very existence to the industrial farming practices that organics ostensibly opposed.

This disenchantment with organics has given rise to one of the more popular genres of food writing and narrative nonfiction in recent years, something we might call "adventures in immediate food." In this genre, a mix of investigative journalism and public diary, writers investigate the operations of Big Food and attempt to develop a more immediate relationship with their own food. The genre's prototype is Michael Pollan's *The Omnivore's Dilemma*, in which the author investigates four distinct kinds of meals by systematically tracing the supply chains leading to each. Purchasing an "industrial meal" at McDonald's, Pollan follows the ingredients back to Iowa corn farms and Persian Gulf oil fields; procuring ingredients for a "Big Organic" meal from Whole Foods, he visits the corporate farms that the chain relies on for vast quantities of organic foods; his "beyond organic" meal is made of ingredients garnered during his week living and working on a self-sustaining family farm in Virginia; and the book's final chapter chronicles the "Perfect Meal," comprising ingredients that the author grew, foraged, or killed with his own two hands. This experiment in self-reliance proved a huge best seller when it was released in the spring of 2006, though it is anything but unique. In the next year, the novelist Barbara Kingsolver, environmental writer Bill McKibben, and Canadian journalists Alisa Smith and J. B. MacKinnon each published their own books chronicling their yearlong adventures eating immediate foods, while *The New Yorker* ran a chronicle of Adam Gopnik's more audacious attempt to spend a week eating only food raised in the agricultural desert of New York City.[11] As a result of these and other books and some popular websites by journalists and food activists

(100milediet.org, eatlocalchallenge.com, locavore.org), *Time* magazine ran a cover proclaiming "Forget Organic. Eat Local"[12] and Oxford University Press declared *locavore* to be the Word of the Year for 2007.

Clearly, if there is a trend in responsible food at the opening of the twenty-first century, it is away from organics and toward locals.[13] And without overstating the distinction between local and organic foods movements, it does seem clear that if the villains in the organics movement were DDT and Alar, that role is played in the local foods narrative by "food miles"—the geographic distance food travels "from field to fork." One significance of this shift from the composition to the provenance of food is that the organic focus on chemicals draws attention to contamination and environmental runoff, whereas the locavore focus on distance draws attention to resources squandered in storing and transporting food. Put another way, organics is animated by concerns over purity, locals by efficiency. If organics exhibited anxieties about pollution, locals seem quite specifically about peak oil. (Similarly, if Locke was concerned that the transfer of energy from the self to the world threatened the conceptual foundations for a social contract, locavores suggest that the expansion of commerce globally threatens the territorial and conceptual foundations for democracy.)

I do not mean to overstate the distance between these two appeals for a revolution in our food supply; the issues and often the principals are the same in either case. Samuel Fromartz's *Organic, Inc.*, for instance, treats locals as (literally) one chapter in a broader movement. But Bill McKibben offers a telling illustration of the distinction. In 1989, McKibben published *The End of Nature*, an early and still canonical warning about global climate change arguing that scientific hubris had facilitated the wholesale colonization of "nature" such that there is (or soon will be) no undomesticated realm with which humans can commune.[14] Fifteen years later, he argued that the same hubris, now wielding nano- and biotechnologies, had destroyed humanity.[15] In each case, the organizing logic was contamination, and the result was a story of (industrial or genetic) pollution. By 2007, however, if McKibben's tune was the same, his emphasis was not. In *Deep Economy*, the metaphorics of pollution has given way to that of spatiality; McKibben is now much less interested in purity than he is in locality; if the threat before was contamination, now it is distance. To be sure, the peril looming in *Deep Economy* is not contamination and the transgression of species boundaries, but environmental collapse due to the exhaustion of the world's oil supplies. Said another way, and again following Douglas, we might see McKibben's earlier books as symptomatic of an anxiety about individual integrity in an age of media saturation and chemical living; his latest book conveys an anxiety about territorial borders in an age of globalization.

There is another significance of the shift from organics to locals. For locavores, the relevant currency for evaluating food systems is not price or environmental runoff, but rather calories. McKibben, for instance, notes how frozen peas burn an absurd number of "fossil fuel calories" in order to deliver hardly any "food calories," and Pollan notes a deplorable exchange rate for organic lettuce (fifty-seven fossil fuel calories burned for each food calorie delivered).[16] This attention to a caloric general equivalent places the literature squarely in the thermodynamic approach to food discussed in chapter 3, raising the specter of entropy and planetary exhaustion while also promising to heal Marx's metabolic rift by linking humans to the earth as similar manifestations of the same primordial energy. This is quite explicit when McKibben and Pollan talk about our industrial food system as essentially a machine for converting vast stores of petro-calories into digestible human food, just as a pastoral food system is a machine for converting solar calories and human labor power into digestible human food.[17] More implicitly, in using calories as the general equivalent, locavores measure foods in terms of how much energy they deliver or squander, and they valuate national diets in the same way that economists calculate deficits and surpluses. Ultimately, locavores argue that the industrial food system, like the bloated U.S. economy, operates at a loss, consuming many more calories than it delivers.[18] The debate over local food is thus of a piece with pressing concerns about global geopolitics—especially the expensive wars in the oil-rich Middle East, the weakening U.S. dollar, and the looming environmental crises of peak oil and climate change.

In this sense, and as I argued in chapter 1, dietary practice functions as a form of biopolitics, such that the ethical imperative to buy local contributes to the health of the body politic, promising efficiency and "energy independence" as well as public health and (supposedly) a stronger national economy. In this light, local is the new organic *not* because organics was co-opted by agribusiness but because the organic ideal fails to address the defining crises of this new century, including environmental and energy crises and also the more immediately political crisis of sovereignty under the novel political formation of Empire and the changing nature of political space. This claim is not alien to the literature. In a piercing critique, McWilliams shows that a locavore diet actually fails to deliver on the promises of energy efficiency and that energy claims are merely a relatively effective proxy for the activists' real concerns: waning personal and national power under neoliberal globalization.[19] (We will return to this claim shortly.) In a much more sympathetic treatment, Wendy Parkins and Geoffrey Craig note that locavorism responds to a breakdown in meaning and identity, by reasserting "the increased value of the specificity of place at a time when space seems less 'grounded' and more 'virtual.'"[20]

The changing nature of space is no small concern. The clear and unambiguous ordering of space has been fundamental to the emergence of modern science, property rights, and governance. Since the seventeenth century, political order has been organized around the establishment and protection of clearly delineated spaces: a separation of private from public space, the division of common land into discrete estates, and the relevant actors in global politics being states (not nations) confined by borders and occupying territories.[21] The ideal of political representation is anchored in the establishment of a fixed population bound to a particular territory over which the government has authority. Alongside regional arrangements such as the North American Free Trade Agreement and the European Union that attempt to forge political alliances around populations sharing *nothing but* location and crude efforts at border vigilantism and "online privacy," the contemporary emphasis on "food miles," the celebrations of national cuisine and regional flavor (i.e., *terroir*), and the ubiquitous refrain that local foods promotes "community" seem clearly animated by anxieties about a breakdown of traditional orderings of space. As Hardt and Negri have argued in *Empire*, what is at stake in twenty-first-century politics is not merely the current organization of governance and sovereignty, but the very notion of sovereignty itself. By extension, what is at stake in local foods is not only particular landscapes and communities but also the very idea of community itself.

Two Distinct Alienations

Alongside the shift from chemicals to calories as the metric for responsible food, the locavore movement has also introduced as one of its primary virtues sociability. For if organics promises healthy land and pure bodies, locavores explicitly promise strong communities with immediate bonds between consumers and producers. Brian Halweil opens his esteemed treatment of the movement by noting how local food economies "build solidarity between farmers and their urban neighbors" and rests on the claim that the movement's appeal lies in its "preservation of the social value of good food in connecting people with each other, their communities, and their land."[22] With the standard refrain that farmers' markets are more sociable spaces than supermarkets, facilitating more numerous and more meaningful conversations, this literature emphasizes not only that local foods build strong communities but also that weak communities are one of the primary concerns of political life today. McKibben, directly but hardly uniquely, argues that consumers are willing to pay a premium for local food precisely because conventional food offers a "surplus of individualism and a deficit of companionship."[23] Clearly, this literature appeals specifically to a loneliness that is presumed to be part of the (sub)urban experience.

Sociability was never a central claim of the organics movement, though that movement did respond directly to an alienation endemic to what has been called a "post-domestic" society in which very few Americans lived on or near farms. Writing more narrowly about animals, Bulliet argues that because "people live far away, both physically and psychologically" from the origins of their food, they have come to experience "feelings of guilt, shame, and disgust" when they think about how their food is produced.[24] That is, the mass migration from working farms through the twentieth century created an alienated and anxious population, eager to assuage their guilt and reestablish their connection to the land via an ethical commitment to things like organic foods and vegetarianism.

This postdomestic guilt, subordinating individual desire to the direction of economic markets, resonates with Marx's metabolic rift and Nietzsche's *ressentiment*. This is probably why Guthman finds an uneasy alliance between social and individualistic values among producers and consumers of organic foods. Promising an authentic relationship with nature, a relationship relinquished in the move to a suburban landscape and a relationship celebrated in a nostalgic model of American freedom, the discourse of organic foods romantically conjures both a world of social and ecological reconciliation as well as one of strong, autonomous individuals. Trading in an agricultural ideal managed by wise stewards responsive to the health and sustainability of the land, the literature conjures a food system without conquest and feeds on guilt about both the decadence of consumer society and the violence of capitalist markets.

Pollan's indictment of the Whole Foods grocery chain turns entirely on his claim that it capitalizes on this guilt with a marketing campaign that conjures a less mediate relationship with the land, even though the grocer relies on the same international commodity chains and regional distribution networks as other supermarkets.[25] While some tie Whole Foods's tremendous market success in recent years to an environmental awakening, an ascetic vision of an agricultural system without cruelty or harm, or just another health-consciousness fad, the real lesson of this simulated pastoral's appeal might be that *ressentiment* is a growth industry.[26]

But the rhetoric of community that pervades the locavore literature appeals most obviously to a sense of place and belonging that is commonly diagnosed as a casualty of globalization. The romantic evocation of community and the emphasis on the significance of locality seems a direct response to the declining relevance of space in an age of globalization. Localism, thus, appears as one more symptom of the political condition of postmodernity, of globalization, or of Empire. For just as David Harvey argues in *The Condition of Postmodernity* that nineteenth-century social theory (Marx, Weber) was preoccupied with issues of temporality because the industrial revolution had fundamentally altered the rhythms of life and the experience of time, the contemporary preoccupation with locality arises from the disruption of space pursuant to recent developments in communication and financial technologies. Established ideas about what it means to occupy or govern a space have been upset by numerous social and technological developments: the creation of nonlocalizable spaces on the Internet, the blurring of public and private spaces by Total Information Awareness and the ubiquitous voyeurism of reality television and Facebook, the blurring of workplace and home by the some 25 million Americans working from home, and the concentration of political power in international finance organizations rather than territorially bound states, to list just a few. And since established political institutions (national sovereignty, representative government, and private property) are all predicated on Enlightenment understandings of fixed borders and reliably discrete spaces, the stakes and disorientations of this disruption would be difficult to overstate.

Locavorism displays an ambivalent relationship to this changing nature of space, simultaneously reclaiming and rejecting traditional public spaces. Alongside an unabashed celebration of open-air farmers' markets, the literature on local foods also conveys a more or less explicit critique of urban space. That is, as I will discuss in the next section, local food carries a notable bias against the topographies and the economies of cities, a bias that reflects a loss of faith in the conventional spaces of politics and thus brings along a straightforward—if muted—retreat from democratic politics. The locavore literature trades in a utopian fantasy of postpolitical reconciliation with both neighbors and the land, a reconciliation that organics sacrificed when OFPA mandated that its ideal be mediated by the state and subject to legislative and regulatory struggle. And so organics fails doubly: first, by failing to speak to the territorial anxieties of globalization, and, second, by offering an alternative to conventional food that was no less implicated in conventional politics. Just as the obesity literature of chapter 4 traded in a presumed distrust of institutional authority, the locavore literature speaks to the specific alienations and anxieties of globalization, from peak oil through national sovereignty, by exploiting a widespread distrust of formal institutions and a deep cynicism about political struggle. Most crucially, the literature reflects a political condition in which it is only in their role as consumers that Americans can imagine political power, and in which the privatization of food corresponds to a broader privatization of politics.

Postpolitical Fantasies

Of course, local economies and even locavorism are nothing new. The locavore literature rarely strays too far from Jeffersonian ideals; when Kingsolver explains that her plan is "to eat deliberately," the reference to Thoreau is unmistakable;[27] and when Halweil, McKibben, and others promise that a local diet strengthens communities and increases social capital by promoting an ethics of neighborliness, it is clear that they have read *Bowling Alone*. The movement's promise of direct personal relations between producers and consumers (as well as subjects and objects), relations that were sacrificed first by industrialization and then by the inevitability of global supply chains, calls to mind nothing so much as the sovereign, responsible individuals that are the organizing conceit of liberal ontopolitics and American political lore.

But such localism often trades in a retreat from politics. Lizabeth Cohen notes how one version of localism—the mass migration to suburbs in the 1960s—was at least in part a retreat into racially and economically homogenous zones that could avoid many of the difficult political issues endemic to crowded, diverse, and aging urban centers. These strategically segregated neighborhoods allowed citizens to erect barriers to entry and develop a narrow conception of "the public good" that included only the members of their specific community and was measured exclusively by the market value of their homes.[28] From the view of these constricted neighborhoods, Cohen continues, it was quite easy to justify the unequal funding of urban municipal services, especially schools, such that suburban localism was not necessarily a veil for racism, but it intensified racially concentrated poverty just the same.

Today, Peter Singer opposes locavorism on precisely these grounds: it legitimates a specific interest over the general one and justifies limiting economic support to an already privileged population that is unique only for its geographic proximity.[29] While Singer's concern is broadly cosmopolitan in its concern that local foods would shut down international grain markets that support third world farmers, Gopnik diagnoses a prorural, antiurban bias in the local foods movement,[30] a bias that is on clear display in Kingsolver's celebrations of country wisdom over urban naïveté.[31] Kingsolver proactively denies that she is valorizing the country over the city, though this denial sits clumsily alongside her repeated mockery of people who cannot identify particular crops and her comparison of her family's leaving their home in Tucson to "rats leaping off the burning ship."[32] Pollan admits that the locavore movement conveys "a deep antipathy to cities,"[33] and it is difficult to read Smith and MacKinnon's locavore diary without noting their growing unease about life in a city, for even though they offer very few of the typical plaints of urban life (traffic, crime, noise), the book's central redemptive trope is a homestead 10 miles from the nearest highway, and Smith confesses that the motivation for their project probably lies in her obsessive desire to own land.[34]

This retreat from the city is just the latest version of a retreat from public life endemic to modern liberalism. But as a response to the privatization of political and economic power under liberalism, it bears a peculiar stamp, removing the vocabulary of political resistance to the private space of the family kitchen. Kingsolver, for instance, enjoying some local ice cream, declares that she "could hear the crash of corporate collapse with every bite. Tough work, but somebody's got to do it."[35] While this is clearly a joke, the rest of her book bolsters the suggestion that the answer to the corporate control of food really does lie in an isolated realm divorced from political life. For not only does Kingsolver's yearlong experiment begin (*literally*) by leaving the city, the detailed calculations she provides at the close of her book are quintessentially bourgeois; though she estimates her year of homegrown food cost "well under 50¢ per meal,"[36] this calculation ignores *the primary costs* of the experiment: land (100 acres in Virginia) and lost income (two incomes, in her household). More than fuzzy math, this represents a characteristic effacement of such properly political issues as property rights and labor markets, an effacement that is only made clearer when Kingsolver visits Italy and introduces Slow Food as a movement founded by "chefs and consumers,"[37] even though it would be more accurate to say it was founded by farmers and communists.[38] Similarly, Halweil's landmark account of local foods explicitly derides "the initiative of well-meaning government officials," and dismisses the importance of conventional politics by identifying a "more diffuse, but potentially more powerful, agent" that can fix our food system: "the food consumer."[39] Halweil then offers a list of subject positions capable of initiating real change: "farmer, restaurateur, politician, banker, entrepreneur, student looking for a career, or concerned parent."[40] The odd presence of "politician" and conspicuous absence of "citizen" from this list may reflect a real or perceived powerlessness, but it certainly exemplifies the trend for consumer activisms to ignore the broader political environment in which consumption happens.[41]

In other words, the specific appeal to locavores to eat foods grown within 100 miles of their homes might be less important than the literature's appeal to a widespread skepticism toward the terms and institutions of democratic governance. The locavore literature speaks directly to concerns about the reliability of governmental representation, the authenticity of culture, and the decline in national sovereignty under the realities of globalization. Like diet literatures discussed in earlier chapters, the locavore literature appeals directly to a wounded notion of trust and a widespread cynicism about formal institutions and collective action.[42] Since 1990, "organic" has served less as a mark of an alternative to conventional food, a circumvention of the institutions of industrial production and processing, than as a legal category subject to frequent and contentious revision by the USDA. For not only is the fact that a food is labeled "organic" prima facie evidence that it is *not* part of an alternative food system (the label signifies, precisely, that the food's producer has been subjected to the certifying process established by the federal government), but the meaning of the term has been a constant source of conflict, with disagreement among producers, consumers, certifiers, legislators, and retailers over whether, for instance, crops fertilized with raw sewage or cows treated with antibiotics when sick can be called "organic."[43] Since OFPA, organic food has been implicated not only in global capitalism and industrial science but also with all three branches of the federal government. The fact that the high cost of organic certification systematically excludes the smallest and often most "pure" producers from selling "organic" foods only exacerbates the movement's enduring skepticism toward the state. Hence the recent calls to eat "beyond organic," and, at my local farmers' market, the handmade signs reading "noncertified organic" that serve as the badge of responsible farming.

As a result, the movement's pursuit of intimate relations with the land has veered toward classically liberal notions of individual autonomy and private property. Though it may be but a curious footnote that the primary retailer of these responsible foods, Whole Foods, remains steadfast in its opposition to the interference of both states and labor unions,[44] Guthman notes that organic farmers have always been "deeply suspicious of state intervention" and that consumers have "occasionally" responded to food contamination and safety scares (like Alar) with "demands for more state intervention (i.e., regulation); [but] more often, they began to buy so-called high-quality food."[45] So it is that Halweil explicitly dismisses the value of state regulation and the unmitigated and ubiquitous heroes of the locavore literature are rogue farmers who eschew institutional support or state assistance.[46]

This skepticism toward state intervention is not anomalous in a culture in which discourses of freedom are increasingly reliant on the rhetoric of the market, in which the rhetoric of citizenship has been largely abandoned for that of consumerism. Nor is there anything new in such a flight from politics; utopian movements on left and right have always promised of a world without conflict (or, at least, without permanent institutions in place to deal with inevitable conflicts). What is particularly interesting in this chapter of utopian literature is how it elevates the consumption (both the buying and the eating) of value-added goods to the level of political action. Typically, this involves a celebration of backyard gardens, farmers markets, or, more ambitiously, Community Supported Agriculture (CSA) in which individuals buy subscriptions to particular farms. In each case, political action involves not mobilizing groups, organizing communities, running for office, or even voting, but rather making a series of ethically motivated consumer choices. The privatization of food begun in the seventeenth century now reaches its apotheosis, when even *politicized* food is shifted away from government regulation toward the household budget, dietary choices, and a valorization of "family" farms. The movement's skepticism toward institutionalized politics informs a retreat from the one institution traditionally capable of (if only periodically interested in) resisting capital concentration: the state. Using organics as a model, Pollan invokes a successful food movement "built by consumers and farmers working informally together outside the system, with exactly no help from the government."[47] The lesson from organics, Pollan suggests, is that government intrusion kills such authentic movements. Noting this tendency, it is hard to avoid the charge that by allowing the economic logic of liberalism to overshadow its political commitments to equality and freedom, by allowing the decline of national sovereignty to take with it political concepts like citizenship and collective action, the locavore movement participates in the conceptual apparatus of neoliberalism.[48]

Of course, the locavore movement promises a food economy that could not be more different from the current concentration of agricultural resources under the likes of Monsanto and Archer Daniels Midland. The local ideal is of decentralized and autonomous family farmers rather than the corporate "factory farms" that currently dominate the landscape, and its practitioners are clearly animated by something like an anarchist moral economy in which "'buyer' and 'seller' form a *community* based on a rich sense of mutuality."[49] But because the locavore literature is dismissive of state action while remaining curiously silent on the issue of wage labor, it seems less anarchist than neoliberal. When Smith and MacKinnon, for instance, speak about small farms as "the last redoubt of a gentler capitalism," what they mean is that market prices tend to be rounded down; they make no mention of labor in this gentle capitalism.[50] Even Pollan, who seems most satisfied when he is visiting and working on farms, rarely mentions the existence of hired agricultural workers. Instead, Pollan casts farms as autonomous spaces where sovereign landholders mix their labor with the land to their mutual benefit; his accounts of individual farmers earning their title with their industry and rationality are straight out of American mythology and even evoke Locke.[51] Alongside his obvious concerns about the treatment of alienated fast food workers, this depiction of the fulfilling labor of autonomous farmers exaggerates the contrast between city and country. With this aestheticization of labor, Pollan intimates that farms are innocent of the alienation and exploitation that drive urban economies.

The problem with this contrast is twofold. First, it is misleading. As Guthman points out, most labor even on the sorts of farms that locavores valorize is actually done by low-paid, itinerant, and abused immigrant labor, just as in conventional agriculture and industrial manufacture. In a systematic study of California's organic farms, Guthman turns up "no evidence to suggest that working conditions and remuneration on small 'family' farms are better than on large 'corporate' ones."[52] More than an unstated assumption that "small is beautiful," the locavore celebration of family farms represents a prototypically bourgeois effacement of wage labor. Pollan, again, barely mentions it, even in his excoriation of these same farms for their duplicitous marketing strategies and their abuses of both animals and the land. More dishonestly, Fromartz profiles the benevolent labor practices at one organic berry farm in California as evidence for the gentleness of this kind of capitalism, though he fails to mention that this is *the only unionized* organic farm in the state.[53]

Second, and related, this effacement of wage labor by the productive power of consumption tends toward the fetishizing logic of capitalism, since it characterizes eating not only as a political act but also as a value-creating activity. In one sense, this may be no different from Marx's "social metabolism" in which consumption is a form of production (since eating produces energy) and production a form of consumption (since farming burns fuel) and in which production and consumption are both but processes of transferring energy from one body to another.[54] Locavores similarly offer a thermodynamic approach to metabolic exchange, evaluating food choices based on their caloric efficiency and rejecting industrial food for squandering so much energy in the transportation and overfertilization of crops. Like Marx, then, locavores evoke a structural parallel between producing and consuming, since both are metabolic transfers of energy, measured in either price (Marx) or calories (Pollan).

But when locavores repeat Marx's move—explaining how industrial agriculture metabolizes petro-calories into steak, and how buying local lettuce produces sustainable farms—their argument cannot be separated from a culture that systematically reduces the responsibilities of citizenship to the logic of consumerism. This same thermodynamic approach to food therefore has a strikingly different effect in Marx and Pollan. In Marx, it illustrates how consumer goods embody exploited labor; in Pollan, it allows shopping as a proxy for labor. In the nineteenth century, it reflected the standardization of labor under industrial manufacture; today, it reflects the reduction of social and political life to market relations. To be sure, Pollan's critique of our schizophrenic industrial food system seems unimpeachable, his ethical call for a more immediate relationship with the energy sources that provide the conditions of our lives seems obviously sound, and his resort to endorsing responsible shopping practices owes to the fact that large numbers of people simply cannot engage in raising their own food. Yet his work inevitably participates in a political condition in which citizenship has been reduced to consumerism, and the very ability to conceptualize political action or individual freedom has been captured by the logic of the market. By establishing the market as the institution through which democratic citizenship can be effected, his argument participates in a neoliberal vogue for subordinating political struggle to market exchange. Biopolitically, it substitutes self-governance and individual choice for more traditional forms of industrial regulation. Most problematically, while consuming local food does produce a market in sustainable agriculture, it also produces *the market* as *the solution* to political problems. By contrast, note how Carlo Petrini, the Italian founder of Slow Food, freely calls consumers "co-producers" in order to highlight the productive power of consumption but finds himself openly disgusted by the "wealthy or very wealthy" patrons of a farmers' market in San Francisco who seem to be buying self-righteousness as much as peppers.[55] The lesson here seems that while Petrini, like Berry, seeks to politicize consumption, the current state of American politics reduces this charge to a significantly more privatized version of consumerist politics—one in which it is the market, rather than the state or even people in their role as citizens, that is called on to do the political work.

Cohen points out that earlier versions of consumerist politics (such as the boycotts at the heart of the U.S. civil rights movement) worked to reinforce social solidarity, whereas the consumer model of citizenship since the 1980s has worked to impoverish traditional models of political action. In particular, Cohen chronicles how niche marketing has fractured and segregated society into smaller and more homogenous consumer profiles with narrower and more personal interests, such that as market activity has come to organize a greater segment of the public imagination it has become more difficult to envision an expansive collective identity or public good. For Cohen, the true irony is that while earlier instances of consumer activism promoted and fostered democratic participation, the success and popularity of consumer activism has corresponded with a steady decline in the most traditional and typical form of political action: voting.[56]

One interpretation of this correspondence is that consumerist politics is a ruse that distracts citizens from meaningful political engagement just as diet promises a measure of individual control precisely because our lives remain in so many ways beyond our control. But a slightly more sympathetic cast would say that the dominance of consumer politics owes to a real impotence of citizens in the traditional arenas of democratic politics. In other words, the point is *not* that locavores alibi capitalism, but that the locavore literature has wide appeal because it speaks to an actual lack of opportunities for political action. This argument parallels recent analyses of other political trends, such as Jodi Dean's assessment of the democratic potential of the Internet and Tim Luke's study of the environmental movement's embrace of "green consumerism."[57] When Dean argues that blogs and chat rooms provide an illusion of meaningful participation in public discourse, and when Luke argues that that recycling does less to stall global warming than to give an individual a sense that they are empowered to change the world, neither simply reduces these strategies to duplicitous redirections of publicly minded energy toward "nonpolitical, nonsocial, noninstitutional solutions" to real problems.[58] Rather, both emphasize that these strategies appeal because they cover over "a more fundamental political disempowerment" that individuals experience under globalization;[59] they offer solace from a recognition that there are, in fact, very few opportunities for democratic action and that citizens are actually quite powerless to change the shape of their own lives. As Pollan puts it, "[s]o much about life in a global economy feels as though it has passed beyond the individual's control . . . But somehow food feels a little different. We can still decide, every day. What we're going to put in our bodies."[60]

These narratives each offer a sense of empowerment in an age in which it has become all but unthinkable that agricultural policy, environmental regulation, or the global trade in information will be subject to democratic control. In each case, these agendas are animated by fantasies of political efficacy as well as postpolitical reconciliation, since they each posit a world in which global crises are forestalled not via representative politics and state regulation, but by smoothly functioning markets actually governed by individual ethics. The narratives of immediate food similarly offer solace from the alienating logic of global capital and the exploitation of farmers by promising responsible consumption through the beneficent and mutually beneficial transactions of farmers' markets and CSA. Finally, the bifurcated nostalgia for both Jeffersonian self-reliance and sixties solidarity that underlies popular approaches to food politics owes to a real loss of faith in the institutions traditionally charged with enacting political solutions. The locavore literature, bypassing representative institutions and heralding direct contact between producers and consumers, does not suggest retrieving a strong social contract, but rather facilitating and embracing an egalitarian social network.

Some Politics Is Local

Perhaps I have overstated the case. Though books like *The Omnivore's Dilemma* endeavor to reconcile agrarian populism with social conscience via responsible consumption, Pollan's more recent writings have recognized the inadequacy of consumerist politics. "Voting with our forks can advance reform only so far," he has since proclaimed; real change demands that people "wade into the muddy political waters of agricultural policy" and "vote with their votes as well."[61] Indeed, Pollan's activism surrounding the 2007 U.S. Farm Bill—the omnibus appropriations bill that is renewed every five years or so and that dictates everything from federal crop subsidies to (therefore) the content of public school lunches—inspired millions of Americans to actually investigate this typically obscure and enduringly impenetrable piece of legislation, studying some very complex and decidedly unromantic dynamics guiding agricultural policy and budgetary process, all toward the end of a responsible assessment of the impossibility of redirecting international agricultural markets and trends without the active participation of states.[62]

Similarly, Guthman identifies significant differences between various approaches to local foods. Most notably, she identifies two types of CSA: one in which eaters pay a nominal subscription fee in exchange for a share of the farm's yield, and another in which eaters invest in the equity of the farm and share its profits, its risks, and responsibilities. The former, which Guthman calls "more common and less radical," is a basic subscription arrangement in which consumers commit to a particular grower; they sacrifice some individual choice of goods, but do not significantly alter their role as consumer. But in the latter version, subscribers really are co-owners in the farm (albeit on a limited basis), and Guthman makes a convincing case that it offers a significant decommodification of both food and land, especially as these farms rarely show a profit and typically depend on land grants for their viability.[63] The common version is benevolent consumerism, whereas the latter, while still organized around consumer activity, compels eaters to take on the responsibilities and risks required of community ownership. The common version strives for a postpolitical network, putting a class-biased air of harmonious exchange on the otherwise unchanged institution of the market; the radical version is self-consciously political, theorizing and enacting a form of collective action that transforms the nature of ownership, citizenship, and control.

The common version corresponds to the terms of liberal ontopolitics, with autonomous consumers exercising sovereign choices. In the radical version, however, the very terms of ownership (and self-ownership) are challenged, suggesting a political arrangement of mutual dependence and vulnerability rather than autonomy and inviolability. Challenging the ontopolitical priority of the sovereign individual and attendant understanding of private property and contract, this approach suggests not just a different distribution of property but a different understanding of what property means, a different understanding of how decisions get made, and a different understanding of how people relate to one another and the earth. Such a radical politics, however, operates with a different set of ideas about identity, authenticity, and responsibility; it risks abandoning ideals like individual and national sovereignty that are predicated on an liberal ontopolitics without offering a coherent or convincing alternative. As a result, and as I will argue in the coming chapter, this potentially radical politics often manifests as a radical ethics, shorn of the difficulty of imagining institutional or collective alternatives without a compelling ontology to ground them.

Of course, engaging with the state comes with its own risks. As Wendy Brown argues, appealing to the state always carries the threat of reinforcing and reinscribing this tremendous site of disciplinary and colonizing power. But as her own analysis of the discourse of rights shows, the risks and benefits of such appeals typically arise from the concrete situations being contested, such that what is in some circumstances "an indisputable force of emancipation at one moment in history . . . may become at another time a regulatory discourse, a means of obstructing or coopting more radical political demands, or simply the most hollow of empty promises."[64] In this current context, the question of relying on or taking leave from the state's power to regulate or reform a food system would seem to hinge on the actual benefits and risks to be expected from this appeal. Here, the locavore solution seems to ignore the costs of avoiding the terms of conventional politics, most critically the relatively unchecked ability of agribusiness to mobilize intellectual property law and free trade agreements toward greater capital concentration and ecological devastation, and also allowing the hegemony of the market and the ideology of free contract to determine the terms of even left-wing political resistance.

In this context, the controversy surrounding the 2007 U.S. Farm Bill is particularly telling. In no small part due Pollan's efforts, this bill was subject to a surprising level of public scrutiny from both activist groups and mainstream media. Critics of the bill tied the structure of agricultural subsidies to global warming, rising obesity rates, the energy crisis, and (therefore) a very unpopular war in Iraq. These claims found widespread public support and few to no counterclaims defending this entrenched series of subsidies. The failure of Congress to take this opportunity to revisit and rework this schizophrenic system that ensures the affordability of Dr. Pepper while raising the relative cost of fresh fruits and vegetables certainly means several more years of unwise subsidies and corporate control of agriculture. The real significance of this failure, however, could be more long standing. Insofar as it is seen as yet more evidence that states are incapable or unwilling to address the environmental violations and human injustices endemic to the industrial food system, it offers yet another reason to imagine one's own powerlessness, and yet another reason to trade a politicization of consumption for a consumerist politics.

6   THE MEAT WE DON'T EAT

THE DISCOURSES OF OBESITY AND local foods examined in the previous two chapters reveal a series of anxieties over individual and national sovereignty stemming from the economic, technological, and political transformations of globalization. In particular, the debates reveal concerns about a powerlessness of individuals to control the shape of their lives and challenges to the institution of national sovereignty that ideally provides a level political representation and self-determination. Both offer routes to the kind of empowerment that is supposedly threatened by vast concentrations of wealth, and both, crucially, invoke a nostalgic version of lived space as a prerequisite for this kind of power. In this chapter, we turn to developments that upset yet another foundational concept of liberal politics: that of the human species. To examine this challenge, this chapter explores one of the most culturally and morally loaded practices surrounding the discourse of species: eating meat.

Americans spend an estimated $142 billion per year on meat.[1] Our relationship to this meat is clearly burdened with issues of culture and wealth, morality and civilization, as well as such sticky political issues as the meaning of rights and the ethics of owning living things. While it is probably beef (rather than apple pie) that is the quintessential American food, and while the rancher rivals the cowboy as the archetypical figure of American cultural identity, the meat industry has grown ever more controversial over the past few decades. Today, it is not uncommon to hear ethically motivated vegetarians describing the rearing and killing of billions of animals annually for food as "a crime of stupefying proportions,"[2] while the deforestation, water pollution, and methane emissions of industrial meat production have become increasingly prominent environmental concerns. Since meat consumption typically increases along with wealth and industrialization, concerns about meat production can only be expected to rise along with the development of Asia and Africa.[3]

Beef, of course, is not the same as meat. Americans have established a relatively stable taxonomy describing which meats are appropriate to eat (cow, yes; horse, no; pig, yes; dog, no), and though this taxonomy of course varies across cultures, the mere idea of eating meat from *human* bodies has long evoked revulsion and been used as a symbol of absolute barbarism. While vegetarian theorists like Peter Singer generate controversy by suggesting a moral equivalence of eating cows or chickens and eating severely disabled humans,[4] Americans remain obsessed with cannibalism—real (Jeffrey Dahmer), fictional (Hannibal Lecter), and allegorical (flesh-eating zombies and blood-drinking vampires saturating popular culture at the opening of the twenty-first century). While the near-universal prohibition against eating human flesh seems fairly unidimensional, the permissive and the restrictive discourses surrounding different kinds of meat each trade in a notion of "the human" that has come under increasing fire in recent years from various angles. From scientific discoveries about species and speciation, to biotechnological innovations like genetic engineering and medical enhancement, to "posthumanist" philosophy challenging narratives of both humanity and humanism, the lines separating the species have been revealed as more porous than previously thought.

In this chapter, I argue that this crossing or blurring of species boundaries animates and complicates the debates about meat, rendering Americans confused and anxious about the assumptions and hierarchies that separate permissible from intolerable forms of meat. I show how some of the recent thinking about meat in academic and popular discourse demonstrates a pervasive anxiety about the status of humanity in contemporary politics. The distinction of humans from nonhumans proves essential to the architects of modern liberalism; it is central in the works of Descartes and Locke, and it is implied in the dominant approaches to property acquisition and human rights. Contemporary debates about cannibalism and vegetarianism, like earlier discussed debates about obesity and locality, evidence a crisis in the terms of liberal politics and, as in the cases of blurred national borders and a presumed erosion of individual responsibility, the borders establishing this order have been aggressively policed. As a result, and like the last chapter, I argue that this particular food discourse undermines the very categories we use to conceptualize politics and so increasingly turns to ethical—rather than political—claims.

Cannibals All!

Though conventional wisdom has it that cultures and species are often classified by what they eat, diet is fundamentally a restrictive (rather than a permissive) discourse. That is, we are defined less by what we do eat than by what we do *not* eat. Muslims and Jews do not eat pork, Americans do not eat horse or dog, and, most broadly, "civilized" people do not eat human flesh or drink human blood.[5] This is such the case that the metaphorics and representations of cannibalism have been a staple of Western culture, typically signifying unthinkable social transgressions. Cannibals are ubiquitous in postapocalyptic fiction—from the 1973 cult-classic *Soylent Green* up through Cormac McCarthy's 2006 Pulitzer Prize–winning *The Road*—always signaling the slide into barbarism in absence of civilization.[6] In George Romero's "living dead" films and numerous other contributions to the popular genre, flesh-eating zombies symbolize "a social order that no longer serves rationalized ends, but has taken on a strange and sinister life of its own."[7] Going back to the nineteenth century, Bram Stoker's *Dracula* evoked anxieties about racial purity and sexual predation through the figure of a blood-drinking vampire.[8] More explicitly, Marx famously describes capital as "dead labor which, vampire-like, lives only by sucking living labor,"[9] while George Fitzhugh defends the paternalism of Southern U.S. slavery against the callous exploitation of industrial capitalism in his antebellum treatise *Cannibals All!*[10]

In his cultural history of cannibalism, Frank Lestringant notes that "Columbus can be credited with the discovery not only of America, but also of the Cannibal."[11] Etymologically stemming from *cariba*, a tribal name from the Caribbean Islands, cannibalism "has played a continuing role in Westerners' construction of what it is to be civilized and its imputation to 'savages' has mirrored the historical geography of successive empires, being variously attributed to early Christians, Amerindians, Irish, Africans, and Polynesians."[12] While Columbus charged these natives with cannibalism in order to brand them as savages, "the cannibal" has morphed from an anthropophagous human into metonymical deviant, characterized by all manner of behaviors from nakedness and sexual voraciousness to incest and infanticide. The cannibal, that is, does not just eat human flesh; the cannibal violates all manner of protocols that characterize civilized behavior. The term thus occupies a prominent position in the history of colonialism and has frequently been invoked to justify the exploitation, domination, or execution of native peoples. Though Montaigne famously argued that "we" reject cannibals because their modes of torture are simply less refined than "ours," and Jonathan Swift satirically suggested that eating human children could solve both the poverty and the overpopulation that was afflicting the colonized Irish in the eighteenth century, such inversion rarely disrupted the dominant colonialist discourse in which cannibalism is the mark of an utter lack of civilization.[13]

As for the actual practice of anthropophagy, anthropologists have presented conflicting reports, inspiring abundant and rancorous disagreement about its prevalence and significance. Culture warrior Leon Kass is clearly relying primarily on his presumption of moral absolutes when he invokes a "nearly universal taboo against eating human flesh" that reflects "the near-universal-yet-uninstructed—that is, natural—intuition of human beings."[14] But the anthropological evidence offers a picture of "human nature" that is much less clear. In a much-debated and hotly contested book *The Man-Eating Myth*, William Arens flatly and aggressively denies that there is any reliable evidence that cannibalism has ever been a significant part of any culture and argues that the discourse of cannibalism has only ever been thinly veiled racism parading as science and providing academic cover for colonial expansion. A survey of the research on cannibalism, he claims, offers "an adequate map of twentieth-century imagination" but not much for accurate historical record.[15] This charge has been directly challenged, of course. Lestringant is not alone in interpreting "the broken, burned and gnawed human bones" found by archaeologists in Provence and the American Southwest as "probable evidence of anthropophagous or necrophagous practices at various periods of prehistory," and he dismisses Arens's work as "crazed revisionism" while lamenting its "considerable popular success."[16] Similarly, Claude Rawson chalks Arens's work up to a "postcolonial guilt and imperial self-inculpation," arguing that in his haste to indict Europeans for their racist exploitation of Africa and Latin America, he has run headlong into an irresponsible denial of the evidence that amounts to a liberal counterpart to Holocaust denial.[17]

Without discussing Arens specifically, Jared Diamond echoes the thesis that charges of cannibalism have often been abused for political ends, but he also claims that modern anthropologists have been reluctant to report evidence of cannibalism for fear of being branded racist by a well-meaning academic establishment concerned about the political manipulations of science.[18] Similarly conceding the archaeological evidence of cannibalism at various times and places, Diamond aims to reveal the racism that presumes to judge as subhuman those who eat human flesh out of hunger, to commemorate dead relatives, or to celebrate military victories. Ultimately, while Montaigne and Swift attempt to invert the charges of barbarism, Diamond merely seeks to protect the reputation and humanity of those slandered by a lingering anthropological racism that condemns a practice without understanding it. In other words, Diamond's work offers a cosmopolitan vision in which the liberal tent might be expanded to include all those who, for material or spiritual sustenance, see fit to consume human flesh.

While the empirical record remains (and, for reasons Diamond identifies, is likely to remain) contentious, it seems safe to agree that identifications of cannibalism remain "sometimes a lie and always an intended defamation."[19] So leaving aside the empirical record, perhaps the more interesting question is not *are charges of cannibalism lies?* but rather *why are such charges so defamatory?* Kass claims that this defamation is effective because cannibalism violates a (perhaps *the*) universal moral code. Given the remoteness of the threat of cannibalism, it is difficult to see why it would retain such a central place in our imagination, however. As Douglas interprets the enforcement of dietary taboos as signals of broader concerns about social order, I aim to show that the discourse of cannibalism does not so much violate a universal moral code as challenge a precious yet precarious border between humans and nonhumans that serves as a foundation for established ideas about identity, authenticity, and responsibility. In other words, eating human flesh (even the protein rich, noninfected, and nonexploited flesh of the recently and accidentally departed) is intolerable because it violates an ontopolitical assumption about human exceptionalism that is essential to liberal political thought—an assumption that has come under increasing fire in recent decades from scientists, ethicists, and philosophers. The cannibal not only violates the species assumptions of liberal political order, but it stands as the embodiment of this violation—a metonymical representation of the crisis of liberal order.

The Human Animal

While the discourse of cannibalism invokes an unthinkable moral transgression as a mark of barbarism, vegetarianism is often presented in the lofty terms of a transcendence of animal nature toward spiritual enlightenment. The vegetarian diet, free of the violence and cruelty endemic to meat eating, often signals mastery of the human appetite and transcendence of political culture. While we earlier discussed attempts to domesticate base activities by concealing animal slaughter and disguising the presentation of meat, here we see a positive transcendence of animal activity by refusing to kill or eat animals and by boycotting one of the most violent and dangerous sectors of industrial capitalism. If cannibals are marked as subhuman for failing to use their conscience to guide their diets, vegetarians aspire to a superhuman status where even the body's maintenance is subject to well-developed ethical, intellectual, or political ideals. This, of course, is precisely why Nietzsche has no patience for vegetarians.[20]

In another contrast with cannibalism, vegetarianism is not particularly rare. While reliable statistics are difficult to come by, a recent study found that somewhere between 2 and 10 percent of Americans are likely vegetarian.[21] This is hardly the death knell of the American meat industry; per-capita meat consumption in the United States has remained quite stable over the past decade (if anything, increasing by a few pounds per year), and it remains nearly 50 pounds per person per year higher than it was in the alleged meat-and-potatoes decade of the 1950s.[22] Still, the 2 to 10 percent figure is approximately double the 1 to 6 percent estimates of a decade ago.

Leaving aside the numerous cultures that have remained largely or entirely vegetarian for religious or economic reasons, one sees in meat-eating cultures three basic arguments for vegetarianism: ethical, nutritional, and environmental. Vegetarian treatises typically marshal all three arguments, but it is difficult to read the environmental and the dietary arguments as anything more than supplements to the central motivating core of vegetarian theory: animal welfare.[23] Ignoring the nutritional arguments, and postponing a consideration of the environmental themes of the literature until the next section, I want to consider here how the ethical appeals of vegetarian literature function as a counterpoint to the condemnations of cannibalism rehearsed in the previous section.

Despite the significant differences between Tom Regan's claim that eating meat violates the moral rights of animals, Peter Singer's utilitarian argument that a vegetarian diet is preferable for its minimizing the amount of suffering in the world, and Carol Adams's feminist comparison of the meat and dairy industries to the enslavement and subjugation of women and people of color, what is consistent across the literature is an appeal to the terms of a political liberalism in which the enslavement and slaughter of animals violates the universal principle of freedom from cruelty.[24] Animals, in these narratives, do not necessarily deserve the same protections as humans, but humans are called on to exercise the Enlightenment values of reason and compassion to elevate themselves from the barbaric practices of human history. Bentham's famous appeal to this ethical regard for animals—"The question is not, Can they *reason*? nor, Can they *talk*? but, Can they *suffer*?"—is ubiquitous in the literature and is used as a reminder that eating meat causes unnecessary suffering in the world and to implicate readers in the torture and slaughter of untold numbers of animals. Implicitly, at least, eating animal flesh appears as just the kind of savage activity condemned in the previous section.

As a result, discussions of vegetarianism end up covering the same terrain as the debates about cannibalism—either questioning or policing the line that separates the human from the nonhuman. Kass explicitly links arguments for vegetarianism and cannibalism to the materialist philosophies and sciences discussed in chapter 3; riffing on the adage "you are what you eat," Kass declares materialism "ethically subversive" in denying "the special place of human beings in the world."[25] Kass takes this comparison to its limit when he actually compares vegetarianism to cannibalism and bestiality, all for refusing to recognize the divinity or uniqueness of the human form.[26] Elsewhere, he makes clear his concern that materialism allows us to treat human bodies like any other tissue, thus legitimating both human cloning and abortion.[27] Despite his hysterical indictment of Darwin for justifying bestiality, Kass seems correct in his suggestions that debates about the permissibility of eating meat owe to disagreements about the meaning of species and that vegetarian literature typically attempts to exploit this disagreement to close the moral gap that supposedly separates humans from other species.

Steven Shapin summarizes that all arguments for vegetarianism— religious arguments, scientific arguments, and philosophical arguments— "inevitably involve basic questions about what it is to be human."[28] For this reason, it might come as little surprise that so much vegetarian literature comes from novelists rather than ethicists or philosophers. Nobel laureate J. M. Coetzee, for instance, agonizes over the arguments for vegetarianism though fictional characters in *The Lives of Animals* and *Elizabeth Costello*; and in a *New York Times* essay considering the novelist Jonathan Safran Foer's recent nonfiction contribution to the vegetarian literature, the reviewer paraphrases Coetzee's Costello in suggesting that "[w]hen it comes to understanding our proper relationship with animals, . . . imaginative sympathy—that is, literature—may be a better guide than cold philosophical argument."[29] As Foer himself puts it, "[t]he question of eating animals is ultimately driven by our intuitions about what it means to reach an ideal we have named, perhaps incorrectly, 'being human.'"[30]

Beyond fiction, this approach of considering what it means to be human is perhaps most visible in the growing academic fields of "animal studies" and "posthumanism" in which students of philosophy, history, literary theory, and cultural studies attempt to "break down the categories and distinctions that have defined how we think about our relationship to everything that is not us."[31] While not all contributions to animal studies promote vegetarianism, the field promotes an ethical engagement with animals that affirms—rather than denies—humanity's animal nature. So while condemnations of cannibalism typically invoke a contrast between the rational people who eschew human flesh and the subhuman savages who fail to use reason to transcend or domesticate their base urges (or the civilized and uncivilized, as discussed in chapter 2), the lodestars of the field (Jacques Derrida, Donna Haraway, and Cary Wolfe) all attempt to root an animal ethics in our connection to and engagement with—rather than superiority over—other species.[32]

This literature confirms *part* of Kass's thesis: not the part that likens vegetarianism to bestiality, but rather the part that claims that vegetarianism often owes to a rejection of inherited ideas about species barriers. Indeed, Derrida attacks the very category of species when he claims that the category of "the animal" reduces nonhuman species to an indistinct mass of beings that can be owned, while Wolfe relies on Derrida to claim that "the discourse of species" takes for granted "the ethical acceptability of the systematic 'noncriminal putting to death' of animals based solely on their species."[33] Wolfe continues that (liberal) vegetarian theory from the likes of Regan, Singer, and Adams remains committed to a conventional idea about species that is predicated on "escaping or repressing not just [our] animal origins in nature, the biological, and the evolutionary, but more generally by transcending the bonds of materiality and embodiment altogether."[34] In other words, it remains committed to the "isolated" self historicized by Bordo, the "somatophobia" critiqued by Grosz, and the rationalist separation of humans from animals on clear display in Locke and Descartes. Posthumanism, by contrast, aims not to realize the project of the Enlightenment by instituting a truly rational and universal ethics, but to question the separation of humanity from nature that justified the imprisonment and slaughter of nonhuman animals to begin with.

Postdomestic Meat

In his cultural history of vegetarianism, Tristram Stuart begins around 1600, when Europeans embarked on a series of passionate debates about the relation of humans to animals, and ends around 1840, when the term "vegetarian" was actually coined and conferred legitimacy and identity to what had previously been a peculiar and idiosyncratic set of dietary choices.[35] Stuart notes a variety of social, scientific, and political upheavals of this period that contributed to the movement, including a bloody civil war in England raising questions about the nature of violence, increased exposure to Indian Hinduism through immigration and travel, and scientific discoveries about the nature and treatment of animals.[36]

Contemporary vegetarian literature can similarly be located in a period of upheaval pursuant to social, scientific, and political developments. Remember John Berger's well-known thesis about the rising interest in animal spectacles such as zoos and circuses owing to the disappearance of working animals from daily life, and Bulliet's earlier discussed identification of a "post-domestic" era where humans, having no direct relation with working or slaughtered animals, develop feelings of shame, guilt, anxiety, and disgust surrounding the treatment of animals and production of food.[37] These feelings have become a common refrain in the literature exploring our relationship to meat. Michael Pollan invokes "an unusual amount of cultural confusion" surrounding vegetarianism and the treatment of animals at the opening of the twenty-first century,[38] while W. J. T. Mitchell opens his foreword to Cary Wolfe's *Animal Rites* with a statement that "[t]he question of animal rights tends to produce a combination of resistance and anxiety."[39] My own experience confirms that undergraduates seeing a video of an animal being slaughtered will invariably respond with horror and disgust.[40] The students seem convinced that it is completely natural to be disgusted by this process, and they seem oblivious to the fact that their reaction is only possible in a condition of postdomesticity. These students surely know where their food comes from, and yet the guilt, shame, and anxiety are clearly evident in their faces, their bodies, and their reactionary (and largely empty) vows to "never eat meat again." This anxiety has only grown more pronounced with public awareness of the terms of industrial meat production. Contemporary meat writing—starting with Upton Sinclair's *The Jungle* and continuing through Singer's *Animal Liberation* and Eric Schlosser's *Fast Food Nation*—has sought to exploit this anxiety, creating "digestive dissonance" so that readers' stomachs are too upset to eat meat.[41]

While vegetarianism is one response to the physical and psychological distance that people feel from their food, another popular response is evident in a literary neoprimativism in which nonvegetarian critics of the meat industry prove their ethical bona fides by killing their own meat. In *The Omnivore's Dilemma*, for instance, Pollan endeavors to "take some direct responsibility for the killing on which his meat-eating depends" by spending a day slaughtering chickens on a family farm and then, ultimately, hunting and shooting a wild pig in the foothills of Northern California.[42] Donna Haraway turns to this very same example, hunting feral pigs in Northern California, when she invokes the "profoundly (and diversely) emotional and cognitive demands individual animals and hunters make on each other" to defend a colleague's ill-fated attempt to roast a fresh kill at a departmental picnic.[43] In the past five years, Steven Rinella has published two books that emphasize the redemptive power of killing your own meat, while essays in *The New Yorker* and *The New York Times Magazine* have each chronicled a movement of suburban families raising and killing chickens.[44] In *Newsweek*, one can read of a "new meat morality" in which consumers commit to using the whole animal, rather than the conveniently packaged select cuts, to pay the proper respect to a felled beast, while veteran food writer Betty Fussell proclaimed that she had "never felt the bonds of creaturehood so intensely" as when she, at age eighty-two, hunted and killed her first deer.[45]

A third response to the condition of postdomesticity is on display in treatment of domestic pets. Michael Schaffer uses the displacement of Americans from farms and consequent anxiety over the treatment of animals to explain the rise of a $43 billion per year industry in feeding, treating, dressing, boarding, grooming, and entertaining pets.[46] With Americans increasingly giving their pets human names and taking them to such previously prohibited spaces as restaurants, hotels, and work-places, these animals are coming to look less like a different species and more like children. For her part, Donna Haraway notes that she had her dog Cayenne certified as a research assistant by the University of California because her university has a ban against dogs on campus, but Cayenne's companionship is "not a literary conceit but a condition of work."[47] At the same time, the world's most famous dog trainer, Cesar Millan of *National Geographic*'s *The Dog Whisperer* preaches a primitive reconciliation with nature, where humans control their animals not through rational manipulation and positive reinforcement but by joining and asserting dominance in the pack. In each of these cases—the "humanized animals" sharing our beds and the "animalized humans" asserting alpha status over their dogs—the line between human and nonhuman is blurred.

If vegetarianism, neoprimativism, and pet fetishism are indeed responses to the condition of postdomesticity, they are also examples of what Marjorie Garber calls "scientific gerrymandering" in which the lines separating humans from animals (and machines) are redrawn "to suit the intellectual politics of the time."[48] But the intellectual politics of our time are not reducible to the disappearance of productive animals from daily life. They also reflect changing understandings of species itself pursuant to scientific and technological developments of the twentieth century. The coining of the word *vegetarian* in the 1840s precedes by just a decade the publication of Darwin's *On the Origin of Species*, which significantly intensified concerns about the moral status of animals by demonstrating that the "the taxonomic gulf between humans and other animals is neither as clear nor as wide as was traditionally held in the West."[49] As authors link vegetarian philosophy to the changing ethical coordinates pursuant to Darwinian evolutionary theory, one also notes the parallel resurgences of vegetarianism and Darwinism in the past decade. Kass also links vegetarianism and Darwinism, suggesting that both present "a false view of human life" that puts us on the wrong side of each and every issue in the culture wars.[50] As legislators, judges, clergy, and citizens argue about the moral status of such liminal organisms as fetuses, stem cells, and brain-dead relatives, one cannot help but notice a tremendous anxiety about the confusion regarding what is and what is not human. Indeed, the field of bioethics has flourished in recent years, precisely because modern technology has created so many new difficult cases.

These anxieties of postdomesticity could only be exacerbated by the "posthuman" turn in contemporary philosophy. Haraway declared decades ago that "the boundary between human and animal is thoroughly breached" and, more recently, that "human genomes can be found in only 10 percent of all of the cells that occupy the mundane space I call my body."[51] Such realizations, Wolfe claims, "[reveal] 'us' to be very different creatures from who we thought 'we' were."[52] They also demonstrate that what is happening in the condition of postdomesticity, in research in evolutionary biology and biotechnology, and in posthuman critical theory is that the species barriers used to underwrite our most basic issues of political organization—from democracy to property—are less certain than what was previously thought. These ethical coordinates, it must be noted, guide not only the use of animals for food but also arguments *against* using animals for food and, perhaps most critically, prohibitions against eating humans. For if the species barrier has been "thoroughly breached," what is the difference between eating a human and a nonhuman animal? Further, if the condition of postdomesticity includes a collapsing "moral gulf" separating cannibalism from pedestrian forms of carnivorism, cultural anxiety and confusion should come as little surprise. Again, vegetarian literature often seeks to exploit this confusion, as when Foer offers his own "modest proposal" that urban locavores who care about the environment should take advantage of a readily available form of protein by eating stray dogs.[53]

With this in mind, it becomes all the more peculiar that, throughout her two recent books about animals, *The Companion Species Manifesto* and *When Species Meet*, Haraway barely mentions the fact that we eat animals.[54] Aside from a rather inchoate chapter on chickens,[55] and a passing critique of "the meat-industrial complex,"[56] *When Species Meet* contains only two discussions of food. In one already mentioned passage, Haraway defends the practice of hunting for food as offering an ethical engagement with nonhuman animals. Haraway calls this "not an easy case,"[57] but because it necessarily bypasses the questions of the breeding, confinement, and care of livestock, it does seem at least *relatively* easy. The other, more disquieting, discussion of food involves a meditation on the eating of a human placenta "to celebrate the bloody materiality of community affirmation in welcoming a baby human."[58] Here, Haraway bypasses the question of cannibalism (the word is not mentioned), noting that the genetic makeup of the placenta seems less interesting than the class-based considerations of whether to cook it and the ethical realization that it was "not food from killed or exploited animals."[59]

Haraway's work thus reveals both the stakes and the opportunities of posthumanism. Considering the placenta, she does not establish a series of ethical coordinates that would legitimate certain kinds of food and refuse others, but rather places us in the perpetual position of ethically encountering and deciding our responsibilities to others. So even as this intensifies our responsibility to others, Haraway admits that it proves incapable of providing reliable codes to guide our behavior.[60] With her argument that particular approaches to killing and eating animals might constitute our greatest expression of responsibility to them casually placed alongside what must be called an implicit defense of ritual cannibalism, the work provokes the kind of anxiety and confusion that Bulliet and Pollan identified earlier. Haraway revels in this confusion, offering not answers to pressing questions about human-animal relations but rather a commitment to "radical otherness." In other words, even if posthumanism does not present the kind of moral danger that worries critics like Kass, it does undercut the lion's share of arguments used to guide dietary choices from vegetarianism to cannibalism. And while posthumanism asks us to abandon these long-held prejudices, it is not entirely clear what the philosophy offers in exchange.

Political Ethics

The contemporary philosophical works being discussed participate in what some are calling "the ethical turn" in political theory.[61] This trend, taking sustenance largely from Foucault's late works and feminist philosophies of the body, has attempted to deal with complicated issues of injustice and inequality not by theorizing economics, power, or organization, but rather by rehabilitating an ethical commitment to otherness that is presumed to precede a democratic political agenda. Like the turn to consumerist politics discussed in the previous chapter, the ethical turn has been criticized for forfeiting a properly political vocabulary about collective action and goods for a solipsistic focus on individual generosity.[62] Supporters, however, argue that ethical commitments are a prerequisite for a willingness to engage in the difficult work required for meaningful political change. As Bennett puts it, "[t]here will be no greening of the economy, no redistribution of wealth, no enforcement or extension of rights without human dispositions, moods, and cultural ensembles hospitable to these effects."[63]

Animal welfare is one of the issues in which the stakes and the opportunities of this ethical turn are on most vivid display. Even among writers who share Coetzee's sense that the exploitation of animals is a "crime of stupefying proportions," very rarely is it proposed that killing animals for food should actually be *illegal*. It is, rather and almost without fail, incumbent on enlightened consumers to stop patronizing the offending industries and go vegetarian. Singer's *Animal Liberation* offers the typical response, invoking "the moral obligation to boycott the meat available in butcher shops" and the imperative "to attest personally to the sincerity of our concern for nonhuman animals."[64] Collective, institutional, political solutions are almost completely absent from Singer's work.[65] More directly, Haraway eschews legal action in support of vegetarianism on principle, arguing instead that what is necessary is for individuals to find comfort in "the never settled biopolitics of entangled species."[66]

Compare this with Regan. In a section of *The Case for Animal Rights* headed "Vegetarianism is Obligatory," he asserts that protecting animals "obviously requires more than our individual commitment to vegetarianism." The challenge, he continues, is "to help *to educate* those who presently support the animal industry to the implications of their support; to help *to forge the opinion* that this industry, as we know it, violates the rights of farm animals; and to work to bring *the force of law*, if necessary, to bear on this industry to effect the necessary changes."[67] But even here, why does Regan say "if necessary"? If vegetarianism is *obligatory*, if animals have *rights*, if killing animals for food is a *crime*, why is invoking "the force of law" such a radical idea to be pursued only if consciousness raising does not work? On the penultimate page of *Eating Animals*, Foer notes that just as we do not have the option to buy untested medicines or children's toys made with lead paint, "It shouldn't be the consumer's responsibility to figure out what's cruel and what's kind, what's environmentally destructive and what's sustainable. Cruel and destructive food products should be illegal."[68] But such claims are rare. In Foer, it comes only in passing (there is no elaboration), in the final pages of a book predicated on helping consumers make good choices, and immediately following a longer passage defending the efficacy of consumer boycotts. Today, even arguments invoking laws seem to have taken the ethical turn.[69]

One way to politicize these ethics, as evidenced by Wolfe's work, is via ecology.[70] In attempting to decouple the struggle for animal liberation from the humanist tendency to ascribe to animals rights, Wolfe tries to show how posthumanism recommends an ecological sensibility that is necessarily hostile to the ongoing exploitations of nature endemic to late capitalism. As he puts it, "posthumanism means not the triumphal surpassing or unmasking of something but an increase in the vigilance, responsibility, and humility that accompany living in a world so newly, and differently, inhabited."[71] In other words, just as the digestive turn discussed in chapter 3 informed a protocommunist politics of universal equality, a posthuman emphasis on interspecies vulnerability provokes a heightened sensitivity to our own fragility and interdependence that is an ontopolitical foundation for ecology. According to Wolfe, exchanging the liberal, humanist ideology of Promethean agency for a postliberal, posthumanist ideology of humility and vulnerability necessarily upsets the capitalist industrial projects so arrogant and heedless of the needs and power of nature.

Even so, Wolfe opens *Animal Rites* by invoking the "ethical and philosophical urgency" of confronting the systematic slaughter of millions of animals per year, and he closes with an entirely inward-looking response: "[A] truly postmodern ethical pluralism."[72] As in the argument for local foods, the activities of markets, states, courts, and other institutions are almost completely absent from this analysis, which can only suggest that what he calls "the *institution* of speciesism" exists because consumers tolerate it. I suggested earlier that the turn to ethics is satisfying because in an age of real political powerlessness, calls for responsible consumption can resonate in a way that calls for political mobilization cannot. I have also talked of the seductive promise of individual power through dietary regulation. The ethical turn in vegetarian theory offers an even clearer example of this move: with hardly any mention of the traditional venues and techniques of radical or even representative politics, it offers inward-looking, personal, and ethical responses to what it takes to be a crime of stupefying proportions.

Posthuman Democracy

More structurally, the ethical turn and posthumanism struggle to speak in political terms because they eschew the dominant political vocabulary. As discussed in chapter 2, political thought of the past four centuries has been organized around the dominant metaphor of a social contract in which identical, autonomous, and responsible beings voluntarily choose their political attachments. The terms of posthumanism, however, reject this abstracted theory of the sovereign self, both implicitly and explicitly supplanting the legalistic representation of society as a contract with a new organizing metaphor: "the social network." This metaphor not only names the defining technological innovation of our age (the Internet, Facebook, etc.), but it also animates the epidemiological imaginary discussed in chapter 4, and it stands as the centerpiece of social theory from the likes of Lyotard, Latour, Bennett, and Hardt and Negri.

Just as the new ontopolitical vocabulary that accompanied the transition from the Middle Ages to the modern era brought along profound anxieties about the order and assurances of an earlier era,[73] much political hand-wringing today can be chalked up to the fact that though the metaphor of a network may well capture the flow of information across national borders and the collapse of space due to communications technologies, it is anything but clear how it might inform political organization and governance. Earlier metaphors of the body politic and the social contract, after all, convey discrete political logics—one of organic hierarchies and interdependence, the other of legalistic and egalitarian consent. But while celebrants herald the network as a leveling force and mode of organization, where any node can connect with any other node, it simultaneously conveys a mode of organization *without power*, and it flounders when encountering institutions with sedimented power structures. In an age of multinational capital and military superpowers, it is fantastic to say the least to describe our society as a network, which means that insofar as political actors approach political action through the vocabulary of a network, they lack the conceptual touchstones for political analysis and are conceptually ill-equipped to engage in politics.

Latour's and Bennett's recent attempts to politicize this posthuman, network approach are both quite revealing in this regard. Both admit that this approach requires abandoning (or refashioning) such classical humanist concepts as speech, reason, and agency. Latour admits that the metaphor of a network fundamentally disrupts these established concepts, that viable network theory would have to "redefine politics and science, freedom and necessity, the human and the inhuman," and that a network ontopolitics denies clean lines drawn around objects, selves, and disciplines and thus provokes a "crisis of objectivity."[74] Bennett, similarly, argues that approaching the world as an "interfolding network of humanity and nonhumanity," admitting that "nonhumanity infects culture" as much as "humans infect nature," makes it "necessary and impossible to rewrite the default grammar of agency."[75] This approach revives the "digestive subjectivity" discussed in chapter 3 and carries serious implications for how we engage the other, partly because it affords nonhuman others a greater level of courtesy but also because it disrupts the liberal conceit that humans choose their own course of action. I will return to the politics of digestive subjectivity in the conclusion, but for now I want to note that part of what paralyzes this approach—part of the reason that posthumanism takes the ethical turn, even when discussing crimes of stupefying proportions—is that while a body and a contract each conveys a political sensibility (the former of solidarity and dependence, the latter of autonomy and choice), the network metaphor lacks any definitive political sensibility. In short, this approach allows us to "reshape the self,"[76] but it offers little guidance on how to reshape the self in a manner that facilitates the effective organization of or resistance to established concentrations of power and inequality.

Part of the difficulty of politicizing posthumanism is that so many of our categories for grasping politics remain anchored in the presumptions of humanism: agency, autonomy, and equality all come out of a humanist tradition that treats individual humans as deserving of particular protections. In which case, as posthumanists violate the humanistic conceits that ground established ideas about democracy—rule by the demos—they are insufficiently attentive to how we might organize political power and responsibility and representation without such humanistic conceits.

Bennett claims that fetishistic attachments to "the human" and familiar notions of agency derive either from a Kantian belief in the requirement of grammar or religious commitment to the narrative of salvation.[77] If this is correct, a certain amount of philosophical critique very well may help us. But Bennett ignores the explanation that I (following both Locke and Nietzsche) have given throughout this book for a lingering attachment to the terms of liberal politics and resistance to the digestive turn: that established political vocabularies, and especially the reified notion of the sovereign self that legitimates a social contract, are cherished and perhaps mandated by a real need to hold agents responsible for their actions. As a result, it seems quite possible that challenges to humanism will also disrupt the various political concepts that depend on these faculties—universal suffrage and representative government, for instance. When Wolfe indicts vegetarian theorists like Singer and Regan for their lingering commitment to humanism,[78] he is inattentive to the difficulty in grounding a commitment to democracy without a conception of the demos—a category of being capable of wielding rationality, speech, and agency. That we all suffer may well be sufficient grounding for an ethic of mutual care, but it seems obviously inadequate as a foundation for political organization.

At the risk of reopening the now stale debates about the politics of postmodernism, it does seem like the political imagination at the opening of the twenty-first century remains anchored in concepts like rationality, autonomy, and democracy that themselves emanate from the core conceits of humanism. Given this, we might see the ethical turn as unavoidable to posthumanism since it might upset very simple attempts to theorize politics. Perhaps we lack adequate concepts for a posthuman theory of *demo*cracy, and so long as our political vocabulary remains anchored in humanism, there can be no *political* critique of humanism. This merely updates a familiar claim from Butler: "To claim that politics requires a stable subject is to claim that there can be no *political* opposition to that claim."[79] The point must be to develop a vocabulary adequate to a posthuman politics, not merely brand as political posthumanism's ethical challenge to the vocabulary of conventional politics.

In the next chapter, I will say more about some of the difficulties of this approach, specifically as the kind of mutual infections of humanity and nonhumanity that Bennett invokes find themselves implicated in a discourse of disgust that encourages a retreat from public engagement. But for now, with specific regard to the debates about species and eating meat, it seems that the problem with posthumanism is not that it is wrong, but that it lacks a viable politics. Insofar as cannibalism and vegetarianism both reveal how our political imagination remains mired in humanism, both amount to proactive strike for or against "the institution of speciesism" by putting into question both the specific placement and the general significance of the border that separates the human from the nonhuman. Together, these discourses reveal more than anything else that though the theoretical edifice of humanism is under siege, we still lack a viable alternative.

Rejecting the ontopolitical grounds of not only liberal capitalism but also representative government, human rights, and personal responsibility, posthumanism jettisons well-entrenched political resources and fails to offer substitutes aside from ethical regard. Posthumanism thus lacks a coherent worldview that would allow us to organize and distribute power and resources and a mechanism by which we could confront the industrial slaughter of animals or violation of ecologies, except, ironically, through markets that actually respond to individual preferences. (Indeed, Wolfe's appeal to an ethical pluralism seems to assume that the market *works*— that it delivers what people want.) But without a compelling way to think about the proper ordering of political affairs attached to some conception of humanity that could embody and enforce that order, the question today is not "socialism or barbarism" but rather "vegetarianism or cannibalism."

CONCLUSION

Democracy and Disgust

> Laws are like sausage. It is better not to see them being made.
>
> —Unknown (though perhaps Otto von Bismarck)

THE PREVIOUS THREE CHAPTERS HAVE focused on how discourses of obesity, local foods, and meat have responded to political anxieties endemic to the disruptions of globalization. Those disruptions were identified as disruptions to ideals of self (in particular, ideals of identity, authenticity, and responsibility characteristic of modern liberalism), space (especially the divisions between public and private and the borders between states), and species (the presumed moral gulf separating humans from nonhumans). The ongoing debates about obesity rates, local foods, and meat each appeal to these anxieties and offer fantastic solutions to them via the placating consumerist logic of individual choice. In this sense, the ethical turn rehearsed at the end of chapter 6 and the digestive turn of chapter 3 both respond to a loss of faith in the sovereign individual at the center of liberal ontopolitics as well as the model of sterilized and procedural politics established in the middle of the seventeenth century. They each respond, that is, to an impoverished model of democracy grounded in the virtues of privacy and representation in which the ideal of the sovereign self is so fragile that the very barriers that pose an impediment to collective living and democratic practice are celebrated for their ability to keep us safe from harm.

One theme of previous chapters has been how hegemonic discourses of food—for example, the characterization of responsible consumption as political action, the biopolitical call to individual responsibility for diet, and the medicalization of obesity—have shifted the terrain of politics from a public and collective domain to a personal and private one. This chapter takes a further step and shows how this privatization of food politics is not merely a piece of a broader retreat from public life but provides a vocabulary for human action that undercuts the impetus to civic affairs and political engagement. In short, it aims to link the privatization of food and its attendant vocabulary of disgust to democratic theory.

While chapter 2 chronicled the difference between a medieval "grotesque" body and a modern "closed" one, this chapter aims to take this chapter's epigraph seriously, arguing that Americans are, by and large, disgusted by the political process—not just because of the presumed corruption and duplicity endemic to national and international sport-politics, but because the kind of exposure truly necessary for meaningful democratic exchange requires an experience of the self and the other that violates the ontopolitical assumptions of liberalism.[1] This chapter links the digestive and ethical turns to describe a digestive subjectivity that is quite different from the rational or possessive sovereign subjectivity of liberalism. Predicated on a recognition of physical vulnerability and mutual dependence, this model of subjectivity rejects the privatizing impulse of liberal politics and has often been invoked in anarchist, communist, communitarian, and radical democratic theory. However, I argue that the popular aversion to this challenge to liberal subjectivity—a subjectivity that, again, is threatened by real currents of political and economic power—reflects a failure to offer a coherent and satisfying alternative that could ground democratic understandings and actions. Disgust, I argue, marks this very real concern about the possibility of the digestive subject being a democratic one.

The Substance of Disgust

One hardly needs to read Freud to know that that the body's orifices have long functioned as sites of profound anxiety. Earlier, I situated some of these anxieties in a reification of the individual body arising from the scientific, aesthetic, and political commitments of liberalism—in the specific exchange of a grotesque for a modern body, the latter of which providing the ontopolitical foundation for a social order built upon a legal and representative "social contract" rather than a natural and metaphysical "body politic." I also presented Hegel, Marx, and Nietzsche as challenging this reified individual for refusing to situate that individual in a set of material relations that make life possible. Most poetically, Nietzsche diagnosed this reified subject as having "evolved that queasy stomach and coated tongue through which not only the joy and innocence of the animal but life itself has become repugnant to him"; confronted with the brute material facts of birth, suffering, violence, excretion, and decay, faced with the very substance of the organic, living and dying, body, this subject responds with "the icy No of disgust with life."[2]

This very disgust has been subject to a surprising amount of scholarly treatment in recent years. Some of the feminist philosophy considered earlier deals at least tangentially with the bodily functions (digestion, excretion, secretion, perspiration, menstruation) that are conventionally held to disgust. But probably the most notable contribution is from legal theorist William Ian Miller, whose *The Anatomy of Disgust* has set the bar for contemporary studies of disgust.[3] Drawing on Elias's work on manners, Miller concedes that the term "disgust" (literally: *dis-gusto*, distaste) is an invention of the seventeenth century. Defining it as "an emotional syndrome"[4] that is marked by "a strong sense of aversion to something perceived as dangerous because of its powers to contaminate, infect, or pollute by proximity, contact, or ingestion,"[5] Miller notes that while the term disgust was never recorded before 1600, "by the mid-seventeenth century English would have a surfeit of terms" to indicate such visceral aversions.[6] This idea of contamination proves essential to disgust, and suggests not just a Hobbesian aversion to pain, suffering, or fear but to a desire to distance oneself from the offending substance whose very proximity constitutes a threat.

Though he uses Elias, Miller draws primarily on experimental psychologist Paul Rozin's clinical studies on what foods (or food-like substances) tend to disgust.[7] While these studies focus primarily on the mouth as a site of disgust, Rozin interprets disgust as "a psychic need to avoid reminders of our animal origins" and finds that it attaches the just as well to various functions that violate the comfortable assumption of human exceptionalism: from biological processes like defecation and decay to sociomoral violations like incest and cannibalism.[8] What disgusts, in other words, are reminders that, despite an ideology of humanism and various faculties that allow us to mask our baser nature, we are really just animals.

Miller, however, broadening Rozin's work to account for various gooey substances that have little to do with our animal nature, argues that what disgusts is not substances that blur the line between human and nonhuman, but substances that violate any one of a number of cherished and orienting oppositions: human/nonhuman, self/other, dry/wet, alive/dead, and so on. What disgusts, according to Miller, are violations of any of these oppositions: decaying bodies that are dead but carry reminders of life, viscous matter that is neither liquid nor solid, and substances like saliva and feces that cross the border that separate the self from the outside world. In short, according to Miller, disgust is a response to things that confound a set of boundaries used to organize our world—"boundaries of culture and boundaries of the self."[9]

Miller defends this interpretation by examining *how* and *when* substances like feces and saliva are typically found to be disgusting. For though feces is the primary contender for a substance that is "universally" disgusting, it is hardly ever considered to be disgusting before it is expelled from the body; when it is safely tucked away in one's colon, one rarely even considers that they are touching their own feces. Similarly, one is hardly disgusted talking to a person with a stuffy nose, though that could change markedly when mucous descends just a millimeter to that person's lip or is expelled into a hand or tissue. Citing a compelling study, Miller notes that while human beings drink their own saliva every time they swallow, most subjects wretch at the very idea of spitting into a clean glass and then drinking even a drop of it.[10] From such cases, and parroting Douglas, Miller argues that it is not the substances (feces, snot, saliva) themselves, but rather the fact that they are *out of place* that is disgusting.[11] More precisely, for Miller, what disgusts is when a substance confounds the distinction between what is me and what is not me. William Connolly evokes this same sentiment: "'Don't pick your nose and eat it.' Who would want to in the first place? It's disgusting. You break one taboo about the relation of the bodily inside to the outside when you pick your nose (though everybody seems to do it); another more visceral one when you eat the proceeds."[12] As Miller sums up the principle guiding this common source of disgust, "once outside, out for good."[13]

This same desire to maintain a distinction between the self and the other is, of course, foundational for psychoanalytic treatments of identity. Mealtime, for Freud, amounts to a judgment between "'[i]t shall be inside me' or 'It shall be outside me'" or "I should like to take this into myself and keep that out."[14] But it is made more relevant in Julia Kristeva's notion of "the abject," which refers not merely to an object of revulsion, but rather that uncanny element that upsets the boundary between self and other. By its very existence, feces draws attention to the permeability of the border between the self and other, thus calling into question the very notion of borders, thus calling into question my very existence as a distinct being, and thus offering an inescapable reminder of our tendency to die and decay. Insofar as the distinctions between self and other and between alive and dead are the very foundations for meaning, the abject "draws me toward the place where meaning collapses."[15]

In response to this collapse, Kristeva argues, the mind creates fetishes, objects presumed to have clean and inviolate borders. The fetish (here: "the individual") becomes "a life preserver, temporary and slippery, but nonetheless indispensable."[16] Though Miller does not discuss fetishism or Kristeva, his work parallels this claim, especially as he focuses on the significance of the skin in the popular imagination: as the container of the self, the skin is called upon to bear the weight of liberal ontopolitics, and blemishes and diseases that afflict the skin (such as leprosy and AIDS) become particularly susceptible to discourses of disgust and moral condemnation.[17] Skin, in this analysis, works metonymically, combining social, political, and scientific discourses about individual autonomy, concealing the unavoidable breakdown of the self and, thus, meaning and order.

In this light, digestive processes seem spectacularly susceptible to the rhetoric of disgust. In the next section, I will explore discourses of disgust and food that have little to do with the physical breakdown and metabolism of stuff that is on display in the processes of ingestion and excretion to show how the vocabulary of disgust informs a political sensibility. But for now, returning to this chapter's epigraph, we can note a widespread disgust at the processes of industrial meat production. In the previous chapter, we discussed an anxiety about the treatment of animals in postdomestic society and suggested part of the disgust experienced at witnessing animal slaughter arises from the distance from and consequent guilt about the practice. But now, note how the slaughter of animals violates the comfortable assumption of morality and transcendence that underwrites our sense as autonomous beings. Certainly, nobody witnessing an animal slaughter could hold that the process is "unnatural." But this violent image could well violate the sense of humanity that underwrites political order; in the killing and eating of animals, we appear not as transcendent and rational creatures, but as mortal beasts subject to all the vulnerability and more of the brutality characteristic other animals. Watching an animal slaughter, we are not the ascetic and peaceful creatures of liberal discourse but rather bloodthirsty and violent conquering animals surviving, as Nietzsche says, through assault, exploitation, and destruction.[18] Cleaned, drained, arranged, and packaged so as to be nearly unrecognizable, animal flesh on display in the supermarket is ultimately transformed from abject reminder of animal nature into fetishized object of consumer capitalism.[19] Hereafter, when eating a sausage one no longer has to confront the fact of human and nonhuman mortality; cleanly wrapped in plastic, the animal flesh represents precisely the opposite: the transcendence of humanity over its animal nature. After decades of this mollifying illusion, how could the crude and exploitative experience of meat production be anything other than disgusting? It is better not to see it being made.

The Politics of Disgust

In what amounts to a friendly rebuke to Miller, Martha Nussbaum's *Hiding from Humanity* focuses less on what makes things disgusting than on the political impacts of disgust. Nussbaum agrees with Miller that disgust is characterized primarily by a concern about contamination—"Disgust concerns the borders of the body"—though her concern with Miller is that he is willing to indulge this disgust and use it as a marker of human development.[20] So while Miller criticizes Elias for overlaying a Freudian framework on his discussion of manners (reading the development of manners as a process of maturation), Nussbaum is concerned that Miller himself continues to herald the tendency to be disgusted by certain things as a measure of civilization. Ultimately, Nussbaum is concerned that Miller's approach is subtly (though necessarily) antidemocratic, as it would admit disgust into policy discussions where it cannot but have pernicious effects.

With a more political and less existential vocabulary, Nussbaum refines Miller to argue that what is at stake in disgust is not so much meaning or order, but rather human vulnerability or what she calls "shared incompleteness."[21] Looking at much of the same evidence, Nussbaum characterizes disgust as a response to our failure to live up to the ideals of liberal ontology; though our political discourse has us as discrete, bounded, and complete beings, we are essentially vulnerable, dependent, and incomplete. The disgusting substances already discussed (from bodily fluids to dead bodies) serve as "reminders of our mortality and animal vulnerability."[22] While (or because!) liberalism imagines a transcendent, complete, and independent being that does not and cannot exist, the failure to realize that ideal stands as a point of anxiety that manifests as disgust. In this, Nussbaum's critique mirrors the critiques of a bloodless and disembodied liberalism rehearsed in chapter 2 and Elizabeth Grosz's diagnosis of disgusting substances as an "affront [to] a subject's aspiration toward autonomy and self-identity."[23] In short, disgust is not a response to scrambled categories or loss of meaning.

Instead, "what we are anxious about is a type of vulnerability that we share with other animals, the propensity to decay and to become waste products ourselves."[24]

In contemporary food politics, the discourse of disgust functions primarily around three issues. The first, as just discussed, is the discourse of meat. The second, as discussed in chapter 4, is obesity. Fat bodies, as Lebesco notes in opening her book on representations of obesity, are often characterized in popular discourse as "agents of abhorrence and disgust."[25] Sweating inappropriately and flabbily failing to maintain a discrete shape, presumed to reflect an inability to control one's appetite, the fat body captures many of the features of disgust already rehearsed. Obese bodies enter the public sphere as reminders of the myth of transcendent individuality, visible reminders of our bodies and their recalcitrance. Animalized as "cows" or "pigs," the obese are characterized as indulgent, undisciplined, or, as Kirkland notes, disabled.[26] These bodies remind us of the power of prerational appetite, and the maintenance of an obese body is read as evidence of a failure to maintain the terms of individual sovereignty—a reminder that is felt particularly acutely when, as discussed in chapter 1, political and economic power wither under neoliberalism. While a century ago overweight bodies might have signaled industrial growth and the possibility of financial accumulation, today they inevitably signal downward mobility and economic decline.[27] Recent theories holding that obesity is literally contagious, that it spreads and contaminates like a virus, further resonate with discourse of disgust and the politics of surveillance. In short, the obese body is increasingly disgusting for its calling attention to the precarity of our established biopolitical order; they are impertinent enough to violate the imperative to self-governance and individual responsibility while also calling attention to the threat of economic power and the fallacies of individual sovereignty and self control. Obese bodies offer an opportunity for self-righteous congratulations at avoiding their fate. But more commonly, as Lebesco puts it, "[t]he fat person makes the ultimate bad citizen in that she or he reveals the American Dream for what it is: a fabrication."[28]

The third domain of disgust in contemporary food politics surrounds genetically modified organisms (GMOs). The biotech industry has in recent years had to contend with what critics call "the yuck factor": the immediate (and arguably irrational) aversion that so many individuals have to the idea of combining genes of distinct species into "improved" lines of plants or animals or, only slightly further in our culinary future, cloning animals and growing synthetic meat in laboratories.[29] As one philosopher puts it in a popular article, those disgusted by biotechnology "are objecting to attacks on *the concept of species*. And in my view there is good reason for that objection."[30]

The most visible and influential expression of the yuck factor comes in an essay by Kass published in *The New Republic* called "The Wisdom of Repugnance." Before taking the helm of President George W. Bush's Council on Bioethics and coming to notoriety for spearheading the council's opposition to embryonic stem cell research, Kass argued that the widespread revulsion to some practices like human cloning represent "the emotional expression of deep wisdom, beyond reason's power to fully articulate it." Directly parallel to his argument about cannibalism discussed in chapter 6, the disgust felt at various uses of biotechnology reflects a "revolt" against "the violation of things that we rightfully hold dear"—more specifically, a visceral reaction to a violation of human dignity.[31]

In fact, Kass elsewhere appeals to this same repugnance in a discussion of the manners chronicled by Elias in chapter 2; talking with your mouth full, licking your fingers, and wiping your mouth on your sleeve are all disgusting behaviors, unbefitting civilized humans. Evoking an anxiety about species barriers, Kass argues that we ought to "[e]at conspicuously and like a human being."[32] Kass specifically indicts carnival foods, like ice cream cones, which require us to extend our tongue into the world to find food rather than using utensils to prepare food and deliver it to the mouth.[33] Such eating amounts to "catlike" or "doglike feeding" that displays a "lack of self control: It betokens enslavement to the belly."[34] Discussing the sensation felt at seeing somebody talk with their mouth full, of having on display the process of food being processed by the body, of world becoming self, Kass sums the principle: "No involuntary participation in someone else's digestion."[35]

But "doglike feeding" is no mere metaphor; Kass means this quite literally. Refined eating—eating at a table, with utensils—"is not so much a transcendence of animality as it is the turning of animality into its peculiarly human and regulated form."[36] Channeling Rozin through his own moral and political agenda, Kass argues that what links the sources of disgust (from cloned meat to cannibalism to licking your fingers) is that they violate a precious-but-threatened border that separates the human from the nonhuman. Disgust is a reminder of our animal nature, a reminder that threatens the very idea of human dignity and civilization. This, for Kass, is very dangerous territory, for if humans are animals, "moral boundaries are up for grabs."[37]

Nussbaum notes that such hyperbolic declarations raise suspicion about the reliability of disgust. Focusing on three *legal* areas that have historically been thick with the discourse of disgust—race (especially miscegenation), sexuality (especially homosexuality), and disability—Nussbaum argues that the disgust does not have a stellar history in motivating admirable or just public policy, as it is easily and frequently mobilized to invalidate or condemn interracial and homosexual relations or to justify treating the disabled as second-class citizens. In light of this history, it is curious to say the least that Kass maintains that the emotion is often a reliable guide to moral judgment.

Cursory examination of the history of racial and sexual policy motivated or justified by disgust offers Nussbaum the clearest case for distrusting this emotion. But it is the discourse of disability that offers her the most theoretical leverage for her concerns about disgust. Nussbaum claims that encounters with disabled (deformed, aged, infirm) bodies commonly elicit feelings of disgust because these bodies force confrontation with the uncomfortable truth that bodies are vulnerable, fragile, and flawed. Of course, insofar as we use eyeglasses or medications, rely on one another for assistance, or grow old and die, we are all, in various ways, disabled. Indeed, the very idea of disability (like Derrida's "discourse of species") is predicated on an ideal of sovereign, fully abled, Platonic individuality that continues to animate thinking about selves and politics despite its manifest unrealizability. In this sense, disgust "is typically unreasonable, embodying magical ideas about contamination, and impossible aspirations to purity, immortality, and nonaminality, that are just not in line with human life as we know it."[38]

But Nussbaum's broadest concern about the politics of disgust surround the very structure of the concept, since its logic of contamination and infection all but prohibits engagement with objects of disgust. Whereas some emotional judgments might encourage engagement or negotiation, disgust (along with shame) operates with a logic of contamination and infection that provokes judgment not only on specific issues but also on any issue that comes into contact with it. These particular emotions, she claims, "are different from anger and fear, in the sense that they are especially likely to be normatively distorted, and thus unreliable as guides to public practice."[39] Irrational fears of the contamination carried in phobic discourses of race and sexuality are well known. But the discourses of obesity and GMOs similarly provoke a moral panic beyond the scope of any reasonable response; witness the readiness to accept the idea that obesity is contagious and the readiness to paint with the same brush crops engineered to withstand drought and human-animal hybrids grown in laboratories. If genetic modification is *disgusting*, that is, we can have no reasonable discussion of the potential benefits of the technology, nor even its political economy. To the extent that we indulge this disgust, Nussbaum argues, we legitimate our desire to hide from ourselves the realities of human mortality, vulnerability, and sexuality. And because the discourse of disgust comes with a logic of contamination, we seek to distance and protect ourselves from things that disgust.

I have been arguing that these things disgust now because of a heightened awareness to or anxiety about the boundaries that organize our lives. This claim, again, mirrors that of Douglas, who ties heightened sensitivity about taboos to broader social disorders. Intolerances for obesity, disability, and biotechnology—conditions and practices that violate the Lockean ideal of discrete and autonomous personhood—reflect a real anxiety about the stability of our ontological foundations for political order. The politics of race, sexuality, disability, obesity, and genetic modification all, like the production of sausage, require intimate encounters with mortal, vulnerable, and corporeal bodies, encounters that threaten the ontopolitical assumptions of the social contract in which abstract and universal, rights-bearing subjects encounter each other in the abstract realm of principle and reason. But the human condition is one of vulnerability, disability, mortality, desire, and dependence. The threatened narrative of the Lockean subject is mirrored in our care for the integrity, unity, and purity of our physical bodies. The disgust felt at so many domains of life today reflects not a natural aversion to threats to human dignity, but an anxiety about the precarity of the myth of individual sovereignty that animates liberal ideology. Alongside Moleschott's and Marx's digestive critiques of individuality, the rhetoric of disgust helps police the borders of the liberal subject. Or, as Nussbaum puts it, "[d]isgust . . . revolves around a wish to be a type of being that one is not, namely nonanimal and immortal."[40]

Hygienic Politics

Previous chapters traced the emergence of a vocabulary of politics that both presumes and asserts the sovereign integrity of the individual body.

Via Locke and Nietzsche, they traced the demand of this ontopolitical fiction to the demands of individual responsibility and representative government. They also argued that this liberal ontology has been challenged by what I called "the digestive turn" in chapter 3 and "the ethical turn" in chapter 6. In each case, the boundaries of the self have been called into question, toward the end of establishing a more harmonious and less objective relationship with a subject's constituent environment. For Moleschott and Feuerbach, this ontological realization opens into the politics of communism. Recent works of Roberto Esposito and Judith Butler help situate this argument in contemporary democratic theory.[41]

While the discourse of hygiene has long been associated with totalitarian politics, Robert Esposito presents the concept of immunity—the legal exemption from any unchosen obligation to others—as "the explicative key of the entire modern paradigm."[42] Esposito shows how political theory since Hobbes has applied this concept to idealizations of the subject with the political discourse of rights being organized primarily around inoculating individuals against the vulnerability to unwelcome intruders. The social contract, for Esposito, constitutes precisely the codification of a relinquishment of mutual obligation and vulnerability and the establishment of a zone of privacy where individuals are immune to the appeals and obligations of others.[43] What I have been saying about disgust can be read as an anxiety about this immunity, as what disgusts is precisely the intrusion of the outside world into the self or the intrusion of a private self into the public sphere.[44]

For Esposito, immunity is the opposite of community—shared obligation and mutual exposure that is precisely the condition that Hobbes's contract is designed to prevent.[45] Similarly, Judith Butler, in her recent works about war and political violence, has focused on the ability to suffer at the hands of another and argues that grief, as a response to vulnerability and as itself a form of vulnerability, gives lie to the liberal myth of the sovereign self. Grief, she argues, reveals "the thrall in which our relations with others hold us, in ways that we cannot always recount or explain, in ways that often interrupt the self-conscious account of ourselves we try to provide, in ways that challenge the very notion of ourselves as autonomous and in control. . . . Let's face it. We're undone by each other."[46] Butler expands this notion of thrall, noting in the next paragraph how (sexual) desire for another and the Hegelian desire for recognition evidence this same dependence. In a "post-Hegelian" vein, Butler chalks up our very survivability to our ability to be recognized by others; we survive not because we are autonomous or sovereign, but precisely because we are, as she puts it, vulnerable—dependent on others for our self-understanding, self-worth, and emotional and physical health. In direct contrast with the sterile politics of the social contract, Butler, at her most lofty, suggests that this "inevitable interdependency [could be] acknowledged as the basis for a global political community."[47]

While Esposito argues that Hobbes inaugurates a tradition of political theory committed to masking interdependency, Miller's work on disgust reveals how the immunitarian logic is just as clearly displayed in Locke, where property serves as a prosthetic body that further protects individuals from invasion from natural forces and predatory neighbors. As Elias measures civilization by the number of transactions made in private, Miller discusses how the acquisition of property and the consequent ability to perform metabolic tasks beyond anyone's sight amounts to a class privilege that only exacerbates the tendency to disgust. In other words, personal property and private space form a buffer zone against encountering objects of disgust (or having others witness your own disgusting acts): "The boundaries of the self extend beyond the body to encompass a jurisdictional territory . . . The size of this jurisdiction varies by culture, age, gender, class, and status. Generally, the higher a person's status, the larger the space within which offenses against that person can take place."[48]

Politically speaking, just as the slaughterhouse hides from us the disgusting process of rendering and grinding animal flesh, the institutions of representative democracy and the extension of so much authority to economic markets shield us from witnessing the processes of legislation and management of public affairs to which we are all beholden. The popular adage linking politics to meatpacking captures this structural similarity; in each case, we take refuge from the practices and activities that reveal our vulnerability and mutual dependence. Broad application of Nussbaum's argument suggests that disgust not only motivates but also actually *encourages* retreat from public life, indulging a longing for a purity, a privacy, or a transcendence that is unavailable in the messy realm of collective living but can at least be fantastically established within the confines of the home. By contrast, a democratically engaged public, for Nussbaum, would be "a society of citizens who admit that they are needy and vulnerable" and are thus more capable and willing to sacrifice and care for one another.[49] Insofar as the liberal subject flees from such corporeal needs and aspires to a realm of pristine autonomy, the discourse of contamination, infection, and purity are not exclusive to the by now well-known discourses of totalitarianism and racism but are endemic to the political philosophy of liberalism as well.[50]

This helps explain how and why food controversies in the twenty-first century offer an approach to politics that is largely restricted to the control over private space. Approached through the rhetoric of disgust, the different questions of animal slaughter, obesity, and genetic modification are removed to a private realm of individualized aesthetic judgment. The retreat from (or consumerization of) politics covered in previous chapters, along with the dietary demands of vegetarian literature, the moral condemnations of the obese, and refusal of biotechnological innovations that question the aspiration to human dignity—each of these phenomena offers a way to manage anxieties about individual and national sovereignty at the level of individual choice. More, they remove political debate of complex issues to the individual consumer, shifting the domain of politics from a public sphere and democratic institutions onto the individual person and their recalcitrant body. Nowhere is this more clear than in Pollan's "protest" and "rebellion" against "globalization" that takes place in suburban homes, on the Kingsolver family farm, or, pyrrhically, through the market.[51]

With the home and body now not only as the site of privacy but also the locus of public efficacy—that is, when the private sphere is not only where one goes to get away from politics but is also the space where politics is possible—heightened attention to the meaning, integrity, and sanctity of that space, and heightened anxiety about the invasion of that space, should come as little surprise. As discussed earlier, scholars have pointed to both anecdotal and scientific evidence to demonstrate that Americans, more so than citizens of other cultures, tend to experience food through the lenses of guilt and shame rather than pleasure or celebration.[52] This could be because, just as the digestive turn calls into question the liberal notions of identity and authenticity, eating itself calls into question the fundamental border between the self and the external world that underwrites liberal ontopolitics; as Latour puts this, recognizing the porosity of the borders around objects and selves provokes a "crisis of objectivity" that Descartes and Locke noted as essential to both reliable knowledge and peaceful coexistence.[53] In a world in which the borders of private space are compromised by technologies of communication and surveillance; the borders of the self are compromised by technologies of discipline, control, and biotechnology; and the borders of states are compromised by immigration, globalization, and terrorism; an inclination to police those borders—via gated communities, personal responsibility, border vigilantism, and localist activism—should come as little surprise. Contemporary trends, in other words, threaten both the narratives of individual and national sovereignty, and discourses of food often reinforce those discourses even as they often (as in the discourse of local foods) would appear to disrupt some of them.

The digestive and ethical turns both serve as rejoinders to the paradigm of immunity, establishing a digestive approach to subjectivity that resists the hegemonic ideal of sovereign or possessive individuality. The dangers of such turns are, by now, well rehearsed: In Hegel and Marx, it tends toward the sort of organic community that cannot help but be intolerant of difference; a return to a preliberal "body politic" that so often allows their names to be heard in discussions of totalitarianism. In Nietzsche, one finds a quasi-vitalist elitism that expresses overt hostility to the democratic sensibility and profanation of the scientific materialists. Butler and Esposito, like the vegetarian theory discussed in chapter 6, forestall some of this difficulty by focusing on vulnerability—rather than any positive attribute like reason or agency—as the foundation for community. That is, if what we have *in common* is dependence, one has the ontopolitical foundation for a humble and generous (rather than hungry and imperialist) res publica. But as evidenced by contemporary expressions of the digestive turn from Pollan, Bennett, and Wolfe, this lends itself readily to an energetic expression of ethical responsibility but few resources for speaking in a more properly political idiom about power, inequality, and organization. This is partly due to a longstanding suspicion about the disciplinary and biopolitical force of such already established political institutions like the state. It is also because the digestive turn calls into question the ideal of sovereignty that continues to be essential to recognizably political discourse.

Butler, for her part, recognizes the difficulty of this radical reimagining of subject, admitting that she does not know how such an approach to vulnerability might organize political life.[54] Haraway, less gratifyingly, announces that her deconstructive work systematically shuns institutionalization and seeks to create and maintain spaces of uncertainty and confusion that would require diligent and constant ethical awareness.[55] But less convincingly, Bennett leaves the reader with comforting assurance that her critique of humanism can indeed be political, and that her extension of agency, speech, and even *democracy* to nonhuman and even nonliving things can indeed promote robust solutions to the climate crisis and can avoid the paralyzing confusion that tends to accompany any troubling of the primacy of the needs of humans over other species.[56] Like Wolfe, Bennett proves inattentive to the degree to which our political imagination is anchored in terms like rights and democracy *precisely because* they offer political expression of the humanist ideal of the sovereign individual exercising agency and speech. She is, in other words, left promising the continuance and expansion of democracy, even as her philosophy itself undercuts the ontopolitical moorings for a valorization of democracy. She endeavors to explain why we can still have it, but fails to explain why we would still want it. In other words, theorists of the digestive turn are left, typically, with two unsatisfying alternatives: maintaining we can retain these crucial concepts even without their ontopolitical moorings (e.g., Bennett), or asking us to welcome a biopolitical condition without those moorings (e.g., Haraway). Either way (and as in Pollan), the best we can muster is individual responses, with little or no recourse to a properly political vocabulary about power, institutions, and governance.

Digestive Subjects and the Twilight of Sovereignty

My point is not that the possessive or the digestive subject can solve the dilemmas of contemporary sovereignty. While liberal, immunitarian politics certainly poses obstacles to a vibrant democratic theory and while I think the politics of disgust reveal those obstacles for what they are, the digestive subject threatens to jettison so many political categories that seem indispensible to a reasonable ordering of human activity. Further, I have argued all along that the anxieties of sovereignty are not fantastic— that the threats to the institutions and concept of political order (especially individual and national sovereignty) are real. Technologies of communication, surveillance, trade, and biotechnology do threaten the viability of such concepts as identity, authenticity, and responsibility. Similarly, the anxieties about powerlessness under globalization are not themselves unfounded; they do seem to represent a real or perceived foreclosure of political opportunity under neoliberalism. The contemporary face of food politics puts it this way: "So much about life in a global economy feels as though it has passed beyond the individual's control— what happens to our jobs, to the prices at the gas station, to the vote in the legislature. But somehow food still feels a little different. We can still decide, every day, what we're going to put in our bodies, what sort of food chain we want to participate in."[57]

In so much writing about food—from locavores and vegetarians, fat activists and diet gurus—concerns about this powerlessness are channeled in to manageable, metabolic programs for individual control. Consumer activity is elevated to political action, control of one's body compensates for control over one's life. When Pollan summons the market as the domain in which to fight out the future of our food supply— we can inaugurate a new food system "with exactly no help from the government"[58]—it becomes clear that these private solutions to public problems are not so much an ideological distraction from the true site of politics, but a biopolitical transposition of the site of politics from the state and public institutions to the individual body. In other words, and what seem to be obvious concession to this in the literature, food politics are not mere distractions from a real powerlessness owing to the shifts of globalization, but are themselves evidence of how contemporary political order is managed through the paradigm of biopolitics as much as sovereignty.

I have also shown how the increased anxieties about food replicate or parallel broader anxieties about the collapse of self, space, and species endemic to globalization. Concerns about these transformations are not wrongheaded or blindly ideological; contemporary political vocabularies—and understandings of such concepts as responsibility, property, and governance—are predicated on received notions of self, spaces, and species. As a result, just as officials and theorists wonder what global order might look like without national sovereignty and individual responsibility, it is not just conservative reactionary politics that worries about the breakdown in the ontopolitics of liberalism with the kind of predictability and order it brings. Just as physical walls along national borders reinforce traditional notions of space and sovereignty even as they paradoxically demonstrate the challenges of globalization,[59] a law insisting that individuals bear sole responsibility for their own obesity reinforces a traditional form of governance *precisely because* that form of governance is proving increasingly untenable and local food activists reclaim the significance of lived and public space *precisely because* it appears so irrelevant to a virtual and capitalized world. Such discourses of food offer a return to a digestible form of social order.

In this light, the contemporary scene mirrors that of the seventeenth century, when widespread disruptions to social and political order created a demand for greater regulation of the borders used to establish that order. Such a homology of individual sovereignty and national sovereignty is, of course, nothing new. In Hobbes, submission to the Leviathan—the "Artificiall Man" composed by uniting the conflicting passions of different individuals—directly mirrors the submission of our own conflicting "appetites" and "aversions" under the power of individual "Reason" to produce the sovereign self. Though our political assumptions and institutions continue to rest on the contractarian logic of consent and authorship, much of the political hand-wringing in political theory and punditry of recent years has turned on threats to this logic in an age of digital communications, online collaborations, international migration, and capital mobility. From debates over intellectual property, to the authenticity of memoir (or the death of the author), to the decline in national sovereignty, to border vigilantism—each of these anxieties owes to a challenge to the hegemonic, autonomous subject of liberalism. Indeed, much of this anxiety could well boil down to a realization that, while political life is more frequently represented in the language of networks than contracts today, it remains anything but clear how the metaphorics of a network might inform democratic institutions.

The political anxieties being rehearsed throughout this book can be consolidated behind the idea that the network is an unsatisfying political metaphor. It does not provide a way to think about power and politics, relinquishing as it does ideas about authenticity and hierarchy as well as territoriality and representation. In this context, one sees a reaction to the digestive turn by policing the borders of self, space, and species in neoliberal politics, local control, and neoprimative attachments to *terroir* and animal slaughter. Contemporary contributions to the digestive turn endeavor to heal Marx's metabolic rift, but such fantastic reconciliations on the Kingsolver family farm or in Singer's vegetarian idyll typically elide rather than contest the global forces predicated on that rift. Similarly, the ethical turn in political theory attempts to mobilize a posthuman ecological sensibility toward better treatment of both humans and nonhumans but thereby participates in an assumption that it is individual choice—rather than bureaucratic inertia and the internal dynamics of capital—that drives the production, distribution, and consumption of precious resources.

The digestive and ethical turns disrupt the politics of individual responsibility and anthropocentric hubris, and they mark a real advance over the sterile, liberal politics of the social contract. But so far, they have failed to offer a viable vocabulary for thinking about politics and democracy, more often than not having rejected the humanist conceits that continue to be necessary for understanding why people would value things like human rights and democratic control. The fact that even these attempts to rethink the terms of politics by reworking terms such as agency, responsibility, and sovereignty tend to revert to that selfsame individualistic notion of individual choice demonstrates the real hegemony of liberal ontopolitics. In writers like Michael Pollan, the end result is an appeal to a society in which markets are driven by ethical—rather than merely profitable—reasoning. In Bennett, we find a disingenuous claim to retain a moderated or tempered version of liberal political ideals; we can have rights, just not a *fetishized* approach to rights. But with this claim, Bennett elides two significant difficulties with appealing to a discourse of rights through her digestive sensibility. First, she ignores the common critique that the discourse of rights does not merely offer a critical form of protection but also produces the very abstract and universal subject that Bennett wants to avoid.[60] But second, Bennett ignores the degree to which the persuasive force of the discourse of rights itself owes to their resonance with the humanist ideal of the sovereign self. Why, that is, would we continue to value rights if we are not humanists? Together, these difficulties amount to a problem of coherence: how can we hang our political hat on the promise of rights if the discourse of rights is as much productive as it is reflective of the liberal ideal of sovereignty? In this sense, the digestive subject wants to have its cake and eat it too—in other words, to reject humanism and liberalism but retain the political virtues that are predicated on humanist and liberal conceits. Insofar as the digestive subject or the social network fails to offer resources for explaining how to pursue freedom *within* this ontopolitical matrix, appeals to these novel vocabularies will fail to offer real productive contributions to the theory and practice of democracy.

In this sense, the terms of liberal ontopolitics remain so thoroughly entrenched in the political imaginary that putative alternatives either resort to those same codes or dissipate into a series of hypothetical abstractions. Nowhere is this clearer than in contributions to the digestive turn. For though these contributions appeal—sometimes explicitly but more often implicitly—to the postliberal terms of Hegel, Marx, and/or Nietzsche, they almost invariably end up invoking some warmed over version of individual sovereignty so as to not disrupt the ideals of responsibility and authenticity that still seem so essential to a compelling picture of human freedom (and still, it must be said, provide very real protections against very real forms of political and interpersonal violence). The revealing nature of food writing in this regard might owe to food being such a nonnegotiable precious resource that nourishes not only our bodies but also our cultures and our economies. Or perhaps it owes to the fact that hardly a domain of human life is not in large part infected with the production, distribution, and consumption of food. Or perhaps it is because food, as I have argued, offers the most intense and material reminder of the mutual dependence of living creatures across the globe. In any event, reflections on food tend to challenge the terms of liberal ontopolitics, thus consolidating and concentrating broader ideas about the meaning of identity, authenticity, and responsibility. Reflections on meat capture deep-seated and uncomfortable ideas about mortality and violence, arguments about Big Food capture concerns about economic power and public safety, and debates about the local farmers' market tap into enduring concerns about the nature and value of public space and the possibility and desirability of those deceptively opaque concepts: community and democracy. If food writing reveals one thing, it is that reflection on eating offers valuable resources for thinking about the value and viability of the terms of liberal ontopolitics. If it reveals another thing, it is that the democratic ethos of food suggested by writers as diverse as Hegel, Pollan, and Bennett is hardly compatible with the dominant terms of political discourse.

While the metabolic vocabulary of food politics opens into a challenge to the hygienic, sterilized, contractual politics of market choices and individual responsibility, it also heightens the anxieties about self, space, and species that are endemic to the transformations of globalization. If disgust is a reaction to the substances that violate the established borders of social and political order (as the discourses of immigration, obesity, biotechnology, and cannibalism suggest), then we can expect to grow ever more disgusted as the political landscape shifts in response to new technologies of movement and communication. The comparison of law and sausage, as things better made in private, both verifies and validates the thesis here about the kinds of selves and the kinds of politics valued in a liberal sensibility. The slaughterhouse, like the state house, shelters us from messy interactions and frustrated sovereignties that are the very condition of political life. The professionalization of animal slaughter, like the professionalization of governance, releases individuals from realizing the real preconditions of their lives. Such institutional protections shelter us from daily recognition that life operates essentially through conquest or that the pretense of individual sovereignty requires repressing our essential vulnerability. In this, democracy is not just like sausage but like food more generally—both fascinating and frightening, something increasingly regulated, packaged, and savored in private but shunned in public. But given that Americans largely distrust both Big Food and the institutions charged with regulating it, perhaps it is time to admit that savoring democracy requires confronting rather than fleeing from the sources of anxiety.

NOTES

Introduction

1 Elspeth Probyn, *Carnal Appetites: FoodSexIdentities* (New York: Routledge, 2000).

2 Michael Pollan, *The Omnivore's Dilemma: A Natural History of Four Meals* (New York: Penguin, 2006), 10.

3 Wendell Berry, *What Are People For?* (San Francisco: North Point Press, 1990), 145.

4 Michael Pollan, *Omnivore's Dilemma*; Eric Schlosser, *Fast Food Nation: The Dark Side of the All-American Mean* (Boston: Houghton Mifflin, 2001); Barbara King-solver with Steven L. Hopp and Camille Kingsolver, *Animal, Vegetable, Miracle: A Year of Food Life* (New York: Harper Collins, 2007).

5 Greg Critser, *Fat Land: How Americans Became the Fattest People in the World* (New York: Houghton Mifflin, 2003); Marion Nestle, *Safe Food: Bacteria, Biotechnology, and Bioterrorism* (Berkeley: University of California Press, 2003); Raj Patel, *Stuffed and Starved: The Hidden Battle for the World Food System* (Brooklyn: Melville House Publishing, 2007); Walden Bello, *The Food Wars* (New York: Verso, 2009).

6 Glen Gaesser, *Big Fat Lies: The Truth about Weight and Your Health* (Carlsbad, Calif.: Gürze Books, 2002); Kelly Brownell, *Food Fight: The Inside Story of the Food Industry, America's Obesity Crisis, and What We Can Do about It* (New York: McGraw Hill, 2004); Daniel Imhoff, *Food Fight: A Citizen's Guide to the Food and Farm Bill* (Healdsburg, Calif.: Watershed Press, 2007); Marion Nestle, *Food Politics: How the Food Industry Influences Nutrition and Health* (Berkeley: University of California Press, 2002); Pollan, *The Omnivore's Dilemma*.

7 Michel Foucault, *The History of Sexuality, Volume 1* (New York: Vintage, 1978), 143.

8 See especially Michel Foucault, *Security, Territory, Population: Lectures at the Collège de France 1977–1978* (New York: Picador, 2007) and *Birth of Biopolitics: Lectures at the Collège de France 1978–1979* (New York: Picador, 2008).

9 See Bryan Turner, "The Discourse of Diet," *Theory, Culture & Society* 1, no. 1 (1982) and Mark Greif, "Against Exercise," *n+1* 1, no. 1 (2004).

10 Pollan, *Omnivore's Dilemma*, 257.

11 My use of the term "neoliberalism" draws on David Harvey, *A Brief History of Neoliberalism* (Oxford: Oxford University Press, 2005), who defines it as "a theory of political economic practices that proposes human well-being can best be advanced by liberating individual entrepreneurial freedoms and skills with an institutional framework characterized by strong private property rights, free

markets, and free trade" (2). See also Wendy Brown, "Neo-liberalism and the End of Liberal Democracy," *Theory & Event* 7, no. 1 (2003), who more pointedly characterizes the practice of neoliberalism as a subsumption of the positive, political rights of freedom and equality under the negative, economic right of free markets.

12 See Martin Jones, *Feast: Why Humans Share Food* (Oxford: Oxford University Press, 2007); Margaret Visser, *Rituals of Dinner: The Origins, Evolution, Eccentricities, and Meaning of Table Manners* (New York: Grove Press, 1991).

13 Leon Kass, *The Hungry Soul: Eating and the Perfecting of our Nature* (Chicago: University of Chicago Press, 1994).

14 Friedrich Nietzsche, *On the Genealogy of Morals and Ecce Homo*, trans. Walter Kaufmann (New York: Vintage, 1967), 253.

15 Nietzsche, *Genealogy of Morals*, 3.16. Hereafter the title of work will be followed by essay and section number.

16 Ibid., 3.11, 3.8, 2.1.

17 Karl Marx, *Capital, Volume 1*, trans. Ben Fowkes (New York: Vintage, 1977), 198.

18 George Lakoff and Mark Johnson, *Metaphors We Live By* (Chicago: University of Chicago Press, 1980).

19 Bruno Latour, *The Politics of Nature: How to Bring the Sciences into Nature* (Cambridge: Harvard University Press, 2004), 22.

20 Stephen White, *Sustaining Affirmation: The Strengths of Weak Ontology in Political Theory* (Princeton: Princeton University Press, 2000), 4.

21 William Connolly, *The Ethos of Pluralization* (Minneapolis: University of Minnesota Press, 1995), 2.

22 See, for example, Emily Martin, *Flexible Bodies: The Role of Immunity in American Culture from the Days of Polio to the Age of AIDS* (Boston: Beacon Press, 1995) and Ed Cohen, *A Body Worth Defending: Immunity, Biopolitics, and the Apotheosis of the Modern Body* (Durham: Duke University Press).

23 Diana Coole and Samantha Frost, eds., *New Materialisms: Ontology, Agency, and Politics* (Durham: Duke University Press, 2010), 16.

24 On transplants, see Melinda Cooper, *Life as Surplus: Biotechnology and Capitalism in the Neoliberal Era* (Seattle: University of Washington Press, 2008); on food, see Brendan Koerner, "Will Lab-Grown Meat Save the Planet?" S*late*, May 20, 2008.

25 See Rebecca Spang, *The Invention of the Restaurant: Paris and the Modern Gastronomic Culture* (Cambridge: Harvard University Press, 2000) or Joanne Finkelstein, *Dining Out: A Sociology of Modern Manners* (New York: New York University Press, 1989).

26 *Oxford English Dictionary Online*, s.v. "consummate," accessed August 27, 2012, http://www.oed.com/view/Entry/39984.

27 *Oxford English Dictionary Online*, s.v. "restore," accessed August 27, 2012, http://www.oed.com/view/Entry/163992.

28 This is true of critics across the political spectrum. For a version from the Right, see Kass, *The Hungry Soul*. From the Left, see Sidney Mintz, *Sweetness and Power: The Place of Sugar in Modern History* (New York: Penguin Books, 1985) or Schlosser,

Fast Food Nation. From somewhere in between, see Pollan's *Omnivore's Dilemma* or Critser's *Fat Land*.

29 Richard Bulliet, *Hunters, Herders, and Hamburgers: The Past and Future of Human-Animal Relationships* (New York: Columbia University Press, 2005).

30 See, for example, Michael Hardt and Antonio Negri, *Empire* (Cambridge: Harvard University Press, 2000); *Multitude: War and Democracy in the Age of Empire* (New York: Penguin Press, 2004); and *Commonwealth* (Cambridge: Harvard University Press, 2009).

31 See, for examples, Richard Sennett, *The Fall of Public Man: The Social Psychology of Capitalism* (New York: Knopf, 1977) and Hannah Arendt, *On Revolution* (New York: Penguin, 1963).

32 See Michael Sandel, *Democracy's Discontent: American in Search of a Public Philosophy* (Cambridge: Harvard University Press, 1996); Lizabeth Cohen, *A Consumer's Republic: The Politics of Mass Consumption in Postwar America* (New York: Vintage, 2004); or Andrew Szasz, *Shopping Our Way to Safety: How We Changed from Protecting the Environment to Protecting Ourselves* (Minneapolis: University of Minnesota Press, 2007).

33 Pollan, *Omnivore's Dilemma*, 254–55.

34 Brown, "Neo-liberalism and the End of Liberal Democracy."

35 For example, Bello, *Food Wars*; Vandana Shiva, *Stolen Harvest: The Hijacking of the Global Food Supply* (Boston: South End Press, 2000).

36 Michael Pollan, *Food Rules: An Eater's Manifesto* (New York: Penguin, 2009); Pollan, *Omnivore's Dilemma*.

37 Nestle, *Food Politics*; Glenn Gaesser, *Big Fat Lies*; Paul Campos, *The Obesity Myth: Why America's Obsession with Weight Is Hazardous to Your Health* (New York: Gotham, 2004); J. Eric Oliver, *Fat Politics: The Real Story behind America's Obesity Epidemic* (Oxford: Oxford University Press, 2006).

38 Barry Glassner, *The Gospel of Food: Everything You Think You Know about Food Is Wrong* (New York: Ecco, 2007).

39 Gary Taubes, *Good Calories, Bad Calories: Challenging the Conventional Wisdom on Diet, Weight Control, and Disease* (New York: Knopf, 2007).

40 Brownell, *Food Fight*; Nestle, *Food Politics*.

41 On agency, see Latour, *The Politics of Nature*; and Jane Bennet, *Vibrant Matter: A Political Ecology of Things* (Durham: Duke University Press, 2010). On responsibility, see Iris Marion Young, *Responsibility for Justice* (Oxford: Oxford University Press, 2011); François Raffoul, *The Origins of Responsibility* (Bloomington: Indiana University Press, 2010); and Chad Lavin, *The Politics of Responsibility* (Champaign-Urbana: University of Illinois Press, 2008). On sovereignty, see Hardt and Negri's *Empire*, *Multitude*, and *Commonwealth*; and Wendy Brown, *Walled States, Waning Sovereignty* (Cambridge, Mass.: Zone Books, 2010).

42 Mintz, *Sweetness and Power*; Pollan, *Omnivore's Dilemma*; Mark Kurlansky, *Salt: A World History* (New York: Penguin, 2002).

43 See Schlosser, *Fast Food Nation*; Visser, *Rituals of Dinner*; Harvey Levenstein, *The*

Paradox of Plenty: A Social History of Eating in America (Oxford: Oxford University Press, 1993).

44 John Talbot, *Grounds for Agreement: The Political Economy of the Coffee Commodity Chain* (New York: Rowman and Littlefield, 2004); Sasha Issenberg, *The Sushi Economy: Globalization and the Making of a Modern Delicacy* (New York: Gotham, 2007). See also Alex Hughes and Suzanne Reimer, eds., *Geographies of Commodity Chains* (New York: Routledge, 2004).

45 Margaret Visser, "Food and Culture: Interconnections," *Social Research* 66, no. 1 (Winter 1998).

46 Levenstein, *Paradox of Plenty*.

47 Lakoff and Johnson, *Metaphors We Live By*. One also sees such implications with terms like "slippery slope," conveying politics as physics, or "the tipping point," which draws on epidemiology. See Dag Stenvoll, "Slippery Slopes in Political Discourse," in *Political Language and Metaphor: Interpreting and Changing the World*, ed. Terrell Carver and Jernej Pikalo (New York: Routledge, 2008); and Chad Lavin and Chris Russill, "The Ideology of the Epidemic," *New Political Science* 32, no. 1 (March 2010).

48 Kass, *The Hungry Soul*, 97.

49 Mary Douglas, *Purity and Danger: An Analysis of Concept of Pollution and Taboo* (New York: Routledge, 1966).

50 Chad Lavin, "Fear, Radical Democracy, and Ontological Methadone," *Polity* 38, no. 2 (April 2006).

1. Diet and American Ideology

1 Historians of diet tend to prefer the terms *slimming* and *reducing* to *dieting*, since all omnivores with even a minimal choice in food sources can be said to be dieting. However, I will be using the term *diet* in its colloquial sense of intentional weight loss plans.

2 Indeed, one of the reasons novel diets continue to proliferate is that ideas about what diets ought to achieve are themselves changing. Some diets promise weight loss, some lower cholesterol, some cardiac health, and so on. Because all diets offer some (incomplete) health benefits (even Burger King's half-satirical and short-lived Angus Diet, which promised greater happiness through greater beefy satisfaction could fairly be seen as providing some health benefits, such as those associated with lowered stress and heightened pleasure), a study parallel to this one would explore not the health risks of cholesterol, but rather how cholesterol came to be accepted as a legitimate focus for dietary literature.

3 Thomas Kuhn, *The Structure of Scientific Revolutions* (Chicago: University of Chicago Press, 1962).

4 John Coveney, *Food, Morals and Meaning: The Pleasure and Anxiety of Eating* (New York: Routledge, 2000).

5 Anson Rabinbach, *The Human Motor: Energy, Fatigue, and the Origins of Modernity* (New York: Basic Books, 1990).

6 Kuhn, *Scientific Revolutions*, 149–50.

7 Ibid., 150.

8 Paul Feyerabend makes the same criticism of Kuhn, claiming that while their ideas "seem to be almost identical," Kuhn maintains the "political autonomy of science" (*Against Method*, 3rd ed. [New York: Verso, 1975], 213). Kuhn, in other words, focuses on the *ideas* or *arguments* that provoked paradigm shifts, whereas for Feyerabend, focuses on the *circumstances* and *events*, "which *cause* us to adopt new standards" (*Against Method*, 16).

9 Max Weber, *The Protestant Ethic and the Spirit of Capitalism*, trans. Talcott Parsons (Los Angeles: Roxbury Publishing Company, 1996); see also H. H. Gerth and C. Wright Mills, "Introduction," *From Max Weber: Essays in Sociology* (Oxford: Oxford University Press, 1946), 61–65.

10 Bryan Turner, "The Government of the Body: Medical Regimens and the Rationalization of Diet," *British Journal of Sociology* 33, no. 2 (June 1982).

11 Nestle, *Food Politics*, 8. Of course, and as I will discuss in chapter 4, Americans do still attribute moral judgments to the overweight, attributing their condition to laziness, gluttony, or some other moral defect. Even so, such critics invariably believe that the ultimate *cause* of their weight gain is a caloric imbalance (rather than a punishment for sin, for instance).

12 Foucault, *History of Sexuality*, 141.

13 Ibid., 143.

14 Foucault, *Birth of Biopolitics*.

15 Cressida Heyes, "Foucault Goes to Weight Watchers," *Hypatia* 21, no. 2 (Spring 2006).

16 Barbara Cruikshank, *The Will to Empower: Democratic Citizens and Other Subjects* (Ithaca: Cornell University Press, 1999), 89, 91.

17 Cruikshank, *Will to Empower*, 88.

18 In *Revolting Bodies: The Struggle to Redefine Fat Identity* (Amherst: University of Massachusetts Press, 2004), Kathleen Lebesco explicitly links the discourse on obesity to the Protestant ethic and the national economy, claiming that "the fat body [fails] to register as a fully productive body in a capitalist economy" (56). See chapter 4.

19 As Marx puts it, "[l]abour is, first of all, a process between man and nature, a process by which man, through his own actions, mediates, regulates, and controls the metabolism between himself and nature. He confronts the materials of nature as a force of nature. He sets in motion the natural forces which belong to his own body, his arms, legs, head and hands, in order to appropriate the materials of nature in a form adapted to his own needs. Through this movement he acts upon external nature and changes it, and in this way he simultaneously changes his own nature" (*Capital, Volume 1*, 283). Marx's approach to both food and labor will return at length in chapter 3.

20 Susan Bordo, *Unbearable Weight: Feminism, Western Culture, and the Body*

(Berkeley: University of California Press, 1993) and *The Male Body: A New Look at Men in Public and in Private* (New York: Farrar, Straus and Giroux, 1999).

21 Bordo, *Unbearable Weight*; Joan Jacobs Brumberg, *Fasting Girls: The Emergence of Anorexia Nervosa as a Modern Disease* (Cambridge: Harvard University Press, 1988); Hilde Bruch, *Eating Disorders: Obesity, Anorexia Nervosa, and the Person Within* (New York: Basic Books, 1973).

22 Bordo, *Unbearable Weight*.

23 Levenstein, *Paradox of Plenty*, 241–45.

24 William Connolly points out other responses to such insecurity, such as hyper-masculine consumerism (monster trucks) and reactionary politics (right-wing radio) in *The Ethos of Pluralization* (113–14). In *Fight Club*—the now-canonical expression of masculine resentment—the protagonists explore two obvious routes to male empowerment: barbaric self-destruction (bare-knuckle fighting) and violent revolution (Project Mayhem). They also offer a summary rejection of another alternative: dieting. Encountering chiseled male abs in a Calvin Klein ad, our hero declares, "Self-improvement is masturbation."

25 Hillel Schwartz, *Never Satisfied: A Cultural History of Diets, Fantasies, and Fat* (New York: Anchor Books, 1986), 5.

26 Ibid., 327. Throughout this argument, it is difficult for anybody familiar with *Capital* to miss that Schwartz is a Marxist, even though he seems to go out of his way not to announce this legacy. Curiously, Schwartz's rather orthodox Marxism has become part of the canon in the fat acceptance movement that I will discuss in chapter 4. Today, even Marxism manifests as identity politics.

27 Coveney, *Food, Morals and Meaning*, chapter 5.

28 Ibid., 73.

29 Irving Fisher and Eugene Lyman Fisk, *How to Live: Rules for Healthful Living Based on Modern Science* (New York: Funk & Wagnalls, 1915), 28.

30 Ibid., 28–29.

31 Lulu Hunt Peters, *Diet and Health: With Key to the Calories* (Chicago: The Reilly and Britton Co., 1918), 24.

32 Ibid., 12. Hoover was not elected president for another decade, but in 1918 he was head of the U.S. Food Administration, the agency charged with coordinating food resources for the war effort. For a discussion of how this fiscal model helped organize the U.S. approach to foreign policy through the twentieth century, see Nick Cullather, "The Foreign Policy of the Calorie," *American Historical Review* 112, no. 2 (April 2007).

33 Schwartz, *Never Satisfied*, chapter 7.

34 No longer a (legal) diet aid, the compound remains an active ingredient in gunpowder and film developer.

35 Harvey Levenstein, *Revolution at the Table: The Transformation of the American Diet* (Oxford: Oxford University Press, 1998), 92–93.

36 Peter Stearns, *Fat History: Bodies and Beauty in the Modern West* (New York: NYU Press, 1997).

37 Amy Farrell, *Fat Shame: Stigma and the Fat Body in American Culture* (New York:

NYU Press, 2010), 27–57. See also Thorstein Veblen, *The Theory of the Leisure Class* (New York: The Modern Library, 2001), 107–10.

38 Turner, "The Discourse of Diet."

39 Michel Foucault, *Society Must Be Defended: Lectures at the Collége de France 1975–1976* (New York: Picador, 2003), 244.

40 Schwartz, *Never Satisfied*, 196.

41 Ibid., 197.

42 No longer a legal diet aid, amphetamines are still a popular treatment for ADHD.

43 Roberta Pollack Seid, *Never Too Thin: Why Women Are at War with Their Bodies* (New York: Prentice Hall Press, 1989), 123.

44 *Time Magazine*, "Fat and Unhappy," (October 20, 1947).

45 See Laura Fraser, *Losing It: America's Obsession with Weight and the Industry That Feeds on It* (New York: Dutton, 1997), 152–53.

46 "Compulsive eating [which is conflated with obesity throughout the book] is an individual protest against the inequality of the sexes. As such, medical interventions . . . are not part of a solution but are part of the problem" (Susie Orbach, *Fat Is a Feminist Issue: A Self-Help Guide for Compulsive Eaters* [New York: Berkley Books, 1978], 193). This argument is still in fashion in the fat acceptance movement (see chapter 4).

47 Jean Nidetch, *The Story of Weight Watchers* (New York: W/W Twentyfirst Corporation, 1970).

48 Ibid., 18.

49 Ibid., 185.

50 Ibid., 14–15.

51 Ibid., 18.

52 Stearns, *Fat History*, 60; John Kenneth Galbraith, *The Affluent Society* (New York: Houghton Mifflin, 1958).

53 Schwartz, *Never Satisfied*, 200.

54 Corey Robin, *Fear: The History of a Political Idea* (Oxford: Oxford University Press, 2004).

55 Kandi Stinson, *Women and Dieting Culture: Inside a Commercial Weight Loss Group* (Newark: Rutgers University Press, 2001); Robert Putnam, *Bowling Alone: The Collapse and Revival of American Community* (New York: Simon and Schuster, 2000).

56 Putnam, *Bowling Alone*, 150–51.

57 Heyes, "Foucault Goes to Weight Watchers."

58 Critser, *Fat Land*, 49–53.

59 Robert Atkins, *Dr. Atkins' Diet Revolution: The High Calorie Way to Stay Thin Forever* (New York: D. McKay Co., 1972) and *Dr. Atkins' New Diet Revolution* (New York: Avon Books, 1992).

60 Barry Sears, *The Zone: A Revolutionary Life Plan to Put Your Body in Total Balance for Permanent Weight Loss* (New York: Harper Collins, 1995); Arthur Agatston, *The South Beach Diet: The Delicious, Doctor-Designed, Foolproof Plan for Fast and Healthy Weight Loss* (New York: St. Martin's Press, 2003).

61 Mark Poster, *What's the Matter with the Internet?* (Minneapolis: University of Minnesota Press, 2001), 39.

62 Fredric Jameson, *Postmodernism, or, the Cultural Logic of Late Capitalism* (Durham: Duke University Press, 1991); David Harvey, *The Condition of Postmodernity* (Cambridge: Blackwell, 1990).

63 Karl Marx, "Introduction," *Critique of Hegel's 'Philosophy of Right,'* trans. A. Jolin and J. O'Malley (Cambridge: Cambridge University Press, 1970).

64 Kuhn, *Scientific Revolutions*, 151.

65 Tricia Gura, "Obesity Sheds Its Secrets," *Science*, February 7, 1997.

66 The term is from Pollan, *Omnivore's Dilemma*, 1–2; the controversial article is Gary Taubes, "What If It's All Been a Big Fat Lie?" *New York Times Magazine*, July 7, 2002.

67 See Critser, *Fat Land*, 50–51; Taubes, *Good Calories*, ix–xii.

68 Schwartz, *Never Satisfied*, 8.

69 Pollan, *Omnivore's Dilemma*, 102–3.

70 Taubes, "Big Fat Lie?"

71 Critser, *Fat Land*, chapter 3.

72 Because the dietary goals established by the USDA in 1977 explicitly recommend *increasing* carbohydrate intake as a means to limit dietary fat (see Nestle, *Food Politics*, 40), skeptics like Taubes have been able to impugn the medical establishment and the federal government not just for promoting an ineffective means to losing weight but for actually *causing* the "epidemic" of obesity. More on this in chapter 4.

73 Stinson, *Women and Dieting Culture*; Heyes, "Foucault Goes to Weight Watchers."

74 Nidetch, *The Story of Weight Watchers*, 18. Discussing other operations that mimic the Weight Watchers formula, Nidetch declares, "It really doesn't matter to me that these imitations exist. I just hope they copy us closely enough so the public isn't fooled and doesn't get discouraged if they join a quack group. Most of these imitation groups . . . give *our* lecture, *our* examples and *our* program" (Nidetch, *The Story of Weight Watchers*, 140).

75 A search of www.weightwatchers.com for "carbs" or "hormones" turns up dozens of such stories.

76 Elissa Gootman, "Weight Watchers Upends Its Points System," *New York Times*, December 3, 2010. This is not to suggest that nobody counts calories anymore. Borrowing from Raymond Williams, we might characterize hormonal and caloric approaches to diet as "dominant" and "residual" ideas, respectively (*Marxism and Literature* [Oxford: Oxford University Press, 1977]). Similarly, the popular literature on "carb addiction" attempted to appeal to the "dominant" psychological paradigm as well as the "emergent" hormonal paradigm. See, for example, Rachael Heller and Richard Heller, *The Carbohydrate Addict's Diet: The Lifelong Solution to Yo-Yo Dieting* (New York: Signet, 1993).

77 See, for example, Schwartz, *Never Satisfied*; Stearns, *Fat History*; or Michael Pollan, "Our National Eating Disorder," *New York Times Magazine*, October 17, 2004.

78 Cruikshank, *Will to Empower*, 88.

2. Eating Alone

1 Visser, *Rituals of Dinner*, ix.

2 These terms, public and private, are notoriously slippery, arguably not as distinct as this narrative will make them out to be, and often complicated by other terms such as "communal" and "collective" on the one side and "personal" or "individualistic" on the other. None of these dichotomies adequately maps on to any of the others, since collectives operate in households, individual interests are expressed in town squares, and collective goods are often pursued in exclusive clubs. More crucially, in *Publics and Counterpublics* (New York: Zone Books, 2002), Michael Warner details how the establishment of a "private" space has long depended on the exercise of a "public" authority, as evidenced by the litany of Supreme Court rulings dealing with reproductive and sexual freedoms that publicly establish a "zone of privacy" around particular acts and behaviors (as much as around spaces). But as Warner also illustrates, there is a familiarity of these terms drawing on widespread prejudices about things that ought to be done behind closed doors versus those that can be done in plain view, and there is often a visceral reaction to the public display of conventionally private acts such as a homosexual kiss, or merely bringing something from one's closet into wide view—that is, "coming out." This chapter continues to draw on what I take to be familiar prejudices about public and private, while their intersection will be taken up in the Conclusion.

3 Quoted in Mark Neocleous, "The Fate of the Body Politic," *Radical Philosophy* 108 (July/August 2001).

4 David Hale, *The Body Politic: A Political Metaphor in Renaissance Literature* (The Hague: Mouton, 1971).

5 Ulrich Preuss notes a parallel and simultaneous shift in meaning of "constitution" in his entry on "Constitutionalism" in the *Routledge Encyclopedia of Philosophy*, ed. E. Craig (London: Routledge, 1998). Originally signifying the empirical body politic (the body is *constituted* by the subjects), the term quickly came to signify the legal charter that organizes the voluntary association of discrete individuals (the legal constitution). "Constitution," in other words, changed from an organic to a contractarian logic. Claude Lefort similarly characterizes modern democracy by its abandonment of the notion of an organic body politic for a belief in universal suffrage, though the logic of a body politic continues to organize the rhetoric and politics of totalitarianism. See his *The Political Forms of Modern Society: Bureaucracy, Democracy, Totalitarianism*, ed. and trans. J. Thompson (Cambridge: MIT Press, 1986), 298–303. Neocleous would seem to disagree, arguing that "the body politic" was replaced *not* with "the social contract" but with "the social body" or "the body of the people"—that is, the population as a mass. However, because this social body was defined not by its metaphysical unity but by its ability to be represented by a government, it still owes more to contractarian than organic logic.

6 Norbert Elias, *The Civilizing Process: The History of Manners and State Formation and Civilization* (Oxford: Blackwell Press, 1939), 43–44.

7 Ibid., 63.

8 Ibid., 55–56.

9 Ibid., 48.

10 Probyn, *Carnal Appetites*, 14.

11 Ibid., 32.

12 Elias, *The Civilizing Process*, 99.

13 This is also, Elias notes, when people stopped serving whole animals at the table, with meat now being cut at a butcher shop or at least in a separate room (the kitchen), so as to remove overt reminders of animal (and consequently human) mortality from the meal (Elias, *The Civilizing Process*, 95–99). This is echoed by Bulliet, who argues that professional breeding and butchering releases individuals from confronting the banality and inevitability of animal life and death, leading to profound anxieties about sex and mortality in contemporary society (*Hunters, Herders, and Hamburgers*). Confrontations with dead animals, and the ethics of eating meat, will be discussed at length in chapter 6.

14 Mikhail Bakhtin, *Rabelais and His World*, trans. H. Iswolsky (Bloomington: Indiana University Press, 1984), 33.

15 Ibid., 281. See also Peter Stallybrass and Allon White, *The Politics and Poetics of Transgression* (Ithaca: Cornell University Press, 1986) or Cohen, *A Body Worth Defending*.

16 That food is more a source of shame or guilt than pleasure in the United States today is one of the points most commonly made in contemporary food literature. See Glassner's *Gospel of Food* and Pollan's "Our National Eating Disorder," for instance.

17 Bakhtin, *Rabelais*, 321.

18 Elias, *The Civilizing Process*, 130.

19 René Descartes, *Philosophical Essays*, trans. L. Lafleur (Indianapolis: The Bobbs-Merrill, 1976), 132.

20 Susan Bordo, *The Flight to Objectivity: Essays on Cartensianism and Culture* (Albany: State University of New York Press, 1987), 8.

21 For more on the development of laboratories in this period, see Steven Shapin and Simon Shafer, *Leviathan and the Air Pump: Hobbes, Boyle, and the Experimental Life* (Princeton: Princeton University Press, 1985).

22 Martin Jay offers a parallel claim that the value of observation and the priority of borders arises from the politics of representation and detachment endemic to a bureaucratic and, more immediately, capitalist sensibility. See his *Downcast Eyes: The Denigration of Vision in Twentieth-Century French Thought* (Berkeley: University of California Press, 1993), 58–59.

23 Bordo, *Flight to Objectivity*, 100.

24 Bordo, *Flight to Objectivity*, 17.

25 Descartes, *Philosophical Essays*, 135. Descartes' phrasing here—"l'union et comme du mélange de l'esprit avec le corps"—suggests that it is as if mind and body were fused (but, in fact, they are not).

26 This mantra is admittedly out of place here, since it was not until 1825 that *ur-gourmand* Jean Anthelme Brillat-Savarin declared, "Tell me what you eat, and I shall tell you what you are" (*The Physiology of Taste, or, Meditations on Transcendental Gastronomy*, trans. M. F. K. Fisher [Washington, D.C.: Counterpoint, 1949], 3) and not until 1851 that Ludwig Feuerbach gave its most literal and lyrical expression ("Der Mensch ist was er isst"). This phrase will occupy much of chapter 3.

27 Elizabeth Grosz, *Volatile Bodies: Toward a Corporeal Feminism* (Bloomington: Indiana University Press, 1994), 5.

28 Descartes, *Meditations*, 132.

29 Grosz, *Volatile Bodies*, 7. Carolyn Korsmeyer makes much the same point in *Making Sense of Taste: Food and Philosophy* (Ithaca: Cornell University Press, 1999). Korsmeyer identifies a hierarchy of senses in which vision and hearing (the "intellectual senses") are elevated over taste and touch (the "bodily senses"), since the former maintain a distance between the subject and the object whereas the "bodily senses" are predicated on a closeness of subject and object. (She places smell in a middle ground.) Korsmeyer roots this discussion in Plato and Aristotle, though she is also clearly drawing on Descartes. Richard Rorty, in *Philosophy and the Mirror of Nature* (Princeton: Princeton University Press, 1999), also argues that though this kind of philosophical purity is often attributed to Kant, its roots are in Descartes and Locke.

30 C. B. MacPherson, *The Political Philosophy of Possessive Individualism: Hobbes to Locke* (Oxford: Oxford University Press, 1962).

31 Grosz, *Volatile Bodies*, 193–94.

32 Connolly, *The Ethos of Pluralization*.

33 John Locke, *An Essay Concerning Human Understanding*, ed. Peter Nidditch (Oxford: Clarendon Press, 1975).

34 Ibid., 341.

35 John Rawls, *Political Liberalism* (New York: Columbia University Press, 1993).

36 Locke, *An Essay Concerning Human Understanding*, 330.

37 Ibid., 331; emphases in the original.

38 See Douglas Odegard, "Locke and Mind-Body Dualism," *Philosophy* 45, no. 172 (April 1970).

39 Locke, *An Essay Concerning Human Understanding*, 331; emphasis in the original.

40 Ibid., 341.

41 Ibid., 342; emphases in the original.

42 Ibid., 343.

43 Charles Taylor offers a similar reading in which "Locke *reifies* the mind to an extraordinary degree" and in which Locke's posited sovereignty fallaciously assumes that "consciousness or self-consciousness [can] be clearly distinguished from its embodiment" (*Sources of the Self: The Making of Modern Identity* [Cambridge: Harvard University Press, 172], 166, 172). For more on Locke's difficulty in identifying a genuine *principium individuationis*, see Michael Ayers, *Locke: Volume II: Ontology* (New York: Routledge, 1991), 215.

44 William Ian Miller, *The Anatomy of Disgust* (Cambridge: Harvard University Press, 1997).

45 Dominique Laporte, *History of Shit*, trans. N. Benabid and R. el-Khoury (Cambridge: MIT Press, 1993).

46 Madeleine Ferrières, *Sacred Cow, Mad Cow: A History of Food Fears*, trans. Jody Gladding (New York: Columbia University Press, 2006).

47 John Locke, *Second Treatise on Government* (New York: Hackett, 1980).

48 Ibid., 9.

49 Locke, *Second Treatise on Government*, 19.

50 Ibid.

51 Bakhtin, *Rabelais*, 281.

52 The bathroom, as Laporte elegantly suggests, becomes the paradigmatic Lockean private space.

53 For a survey of this relationship, see the introduction to James Martel, *Subverting the Leviathan: Reading Hobbes as a Radical Democrat* (New York: Columbia University Press, 2007). Oddly, Hale's study of the metaphor of a body politic in early modern England makes no mention of Hobbes until the final three pages. This might seem an unforgiveable neglect, though Hale might point out that his study ends in 1649 and Hobbes's *Leviathan* was not published until 1651 and *De Corpore* in 1655. I see Hale's omission primarily as indicative of Hobbes's tenuous position in the history of liberalism.

54 Thomas Hobbes, *Leviathan*, ed. C. B. MacPherson (New York: Penguin 1968), 81.

55 Ibid., 295.

56 Ibid., 301.

57 Ibid., 220.

58 Ibid., 161.

59 Again, if the body politic unifies a population through the logic of incorporation, the social contract does it through the logic of representation (Lefort, *Political Forms of Modern Society*, 302–3).

60 Hobbes, *Leviathan*, 689.

61 Samantha Frost, *Lessons from a Materialist Thinker: Hobbesian Reflections on Ethics and Politics* (Stanford: Stanford University Press, 2008), 20–25. For a very different, but ultimately complementary, argument that Cartesian prejudices loom large in philosophies that never admit it, see Jay, *Downcast Eyes*, chapter 5.

62 Thomas Hobbes, *De Corpore*, in *The English Works of Thomas Hobbes of Malmesbury*, ed. W. Molesworth, vol. 1 (London: John Bohn, 1966), chapter 11.

63 Ibid., 137. See also Yves Charles Zarka, "First Philosophy and the Foundations of Science," in *The Cambridge Companion to Hobbes*, ed. T. Sorell (Cambridge: Cambridge University Press, 1996).

64 Hobbes, *Leviathan*, chapter 6; *De Corpore*, 34.

65 *De Corpore*, 501–8.

66 This point is consistent with very different approaches to Hobbes—from MacPherson's claim (i.e., for Hobbes, we own our bodies) to Martel's claim (i.e., "for Hobbes, we simply *are* our bodies"; Martel, "The Radical Promise of Thomas Hobbes: The

Road Not Taken in Liberal Theory," *Theory & Event* 4, no. 2 [2000], section 61). It is *not* consistent with Frost's claim that Hobbes "dismant[les] the myth of the self-sovereign individual" (*Lessons from a Materialist Thinker*, 12). But this is, as we will see, because Frost imputes her own theory of intersubjective ethics onto an unwitting Hobbes.

67 MacPherson, *Possessive Individualism*.

68 Leo Strauss, *The Political Philosophy of Hobbes: Its Basis and Its Genesis*, trans. E. Sinclair (Oxford: Oxford University Press, 1936).

69 Samantha Frost, "Reading the Body: Hobbes, Body Politics, and the Vocation of Political Theory," in *Vocations of Political Theory*, ed. Jason Frank and John Tambornino (Minneapolis: University of Minnesota Press, 2000).

70 Frost goes into these readings in great detail; I presume they are familiar enough for present purposes. To be clear, the point is *not* that Hobbesians actively manipulate Hobbes's legacy for their own benefit, but only that the prejudices of liberalism lead readers and interpreters to focus on particular aspects. This is what I take MacPherson to be saying when he says that Hobbes "more or less consciously" assumes market principles in designing his state of nature, or David Gauthier to mean when he discusses "The Social Contract as Ideology" (*Philosophy and Public Affairs* 6, no. 2 [Winter 1977]).

71 Frost, *Lessons from a Materialist Thinker*, 2.

72 On page 3, Frost directs the reader to Teresa Brennan, William Connolly, Elizabeth Grosz, and Brian Massumi. This influence is also explicit in the introduction to Coole and Frost's *New Materialisms*.

73 Shapin and Shafer, *Leviathan and the Air Pump*; Bruno Latour, *We Have Never Been Modern*, trans. Catherine Porter (Cambridge, MA: Harvard University Press, 1993).

74 MacPherson, *Possessive Individualism*.

75 Sheldon Wolin, *Politics and Vision* (Boston: Little, Brown, 1960); Roberto Esposito, *Communitas: The Origin and Destiny of Community*, trans. T. Campbell (Stanford: Stanford University Press, 2010).

76 Locke, *De Corpore*, 506–8.

77 Strauss, *Political Philosophy of Hobbes*, 5.

78 Wolin, *Politics and Vision*; Esposito, *Communitas*; Judith Shklar, *Ordinary Vices* (Cambridge: Harvard University Press, 1984).

79 Roland Barthes, "Toward a Psychosociology of Contemporary Food Consumption" in *Food and Culture: A Reader*, ed. Carole Counihan and Penny Van Esterik (New York: Routledge, 1997); Claude Lévi-Strauss, *The Raw and the Cooked*, trans. J. and D. Weightman (New York: Harper & Row, 1969); Douglas, *Purity and Danger*.

80 Douglas, *Purity and Danger*, 157.

81 Ibid., 150.

82 See Lefort, *Political Forms of Modern Society*.

83 See Brown, *Walled States*.

84 Richard Flathman, *Thomas Hobbes: Skepticism, Individuality and Chastened Politics* (Newbury Park, Calif.: Sage Publications, 1993), 127n14.

3. The Digestive Turn in Political Thought

1 Again, see Hale, *Body Politic*; Lefort, *Political Forms of Modern Society*; or Preuss, "Constitutionalism." The impact of this sterility will be the focus of chapter 7.

2 Welfare state liberals like Michael Moore often cast their grievances in terms of a broken social contract, while Newt Gingrich promised to renew politics in 1994 with his "Contract With America." The Tea Party, in 2010, tried to revise Gingrich with its own "Contract From America."

3 Pollan, *Omnivore's Dilemma*, 23. This argument is explicit in *The Omnivore's Dilemma*, but it is the central thesis of his earlier *The Botany of Desire: A Plant's-Eye View of the World* (New York: Random House, 2001).

4 Alfred Tauber, *The Immune Self: Theory or Metaphor?* (Cambridge: Cambridge University Press, 1994), 13.

5 Alfred Tauber, "Introduction: Speculations Concerning the Origins of Self," in *Organism and the Origins of Self*, ed. Alfred Tauber (Boston: Kluwer Academic Publishers, 1991), 27. Of course, this is only a challenge to Locke if we read "self" as "body," which Locke clearly does not. But quotes likes this, as well as the challenges to Locke rehearsed in chapter 1, suggest that Locke remains rather unconvincing on this point. Further, current and frenzied political (which is not to say scientific) opposition to vaccinating infants or teaching Darwinism in schools seems to indicate a realization that Darwin's theory of evolution *does* pose a radical challenge to the ideological structures of contemporary political life.

6 It is impossible to determine the exact date of discovery of these principles, but Hermann von Helmholtz's 1847 lecture "Die Erhaltung der Kraft" ("The Conservation of Force") is typically taken as a bellwether. See William Coleman, *Biology in the Nineteenth Century: Problems of Form, Function, and Transformation* (New York: Wiley, 1971); Frederick Gregory, *Scientific Materialism in Nineteenth Century Germany* (Boston: D. Reidel Publishing, 1977); and Rabinbach, *Human Motor*.

7 Thomas Kuhn, "Energy Conservation as an Example of Simultaneous Discovery," in *Critical Problems in the History of Science*, ed. Marshall Clagett (Madison: University of Wisconsin Press, 1959); Kuhn, *Scientific Revolutions*.

8 Amy Wendling, *Karl Marx on Technology and Alienation* (New York: Palgrave Macmillan, 2009), 75.

9 Everett Mendelsohn, "Revolution and Reduction: The Sociology of Methodological and Philosophical Concerns in Nineteenth Century Biology," in *The Interaction Between Science and Philosophy*, ed. Yehuda Elkana (Atlantic Highlands, N.J.: Humanities Press, 1974), 413.

10 Silke-Maria Weinek, "Digesting the Nineteenth Century: Nietzsche and the Stomach of Modernity," *Romanticism* 12, no. 1 (2006), 37.

11 Coleman, *Biology in the Nineteenth Century*, 131.

12 See Rabinbach, *Human Motor*, 66–67, 125–27.

13 Not coincidentally, it was Leibig who, in 1840, first calculated soil fertility as a function of nitrogen, phosphorous, and potassium—a calculation that still governs the production of industrial fertilizers (see Pollan, *Omnivore's Dilemma*, 146).

14 Gregory, *Scientific Materialism*, 88.

15 Quoted in Gregory, *Scientific Materialism*, 89.

16 Locke, *An Essay Concerning Human Understanding*, 331.

17 Gregory suggests that Feuerbach's reputation as a vulgar materialist might be attributed to his being overly excited by the power of Moleschott's book; caught up in the promise of its argument, he forfeited some of his more reasonable senses (Gregory, *Scientific Materialism*, 91–92). See also Melvin Cherno, "Feuerbach's 'Man Is What He Eats': A Rectification," *Journal of the History of Ideas* 24, no. 3 (July–September 1963).

18 At the extreme, Platonic bioethicist and presidential advisor Leon Kass blames this materialism for denying the existence of a soul, refusing the divinity of the human form, and thus justifying both abortion and cannibalism. See chapter 6.

19 Gregory, *Scientific Materialism*, 94.

20 Ibid., 93.

21 Ibid., 95–96.

22 Ibid., 105.

23 Ludwig Büchner, *Force and Matter, or, Principles of the Natural Order of the Universe* (New York: P. Eckler, 1920), 17–18.

24 Nietzsche, *Genealogy of Morals*, 1.13. For a pointed discussion of this passage in Nietzsche, see Judith Butler, *Giving an Account of Oneself* (New York: Fordham University Press, 2005), 14–15.

25 It is surely no coincidence that these materialists championed Darwin's work in Germany or that Marx considered dedicating *Capital* to Darwin (Gregory, *Scientific Materialism*, 186).

26 Coleman, *Biology in the Nineteenth Century*, 111–12.

27 Compare Wolin's characterization of liberalism as "pure" and "sterile" (*Politics and Vision*, chapter 9) with Brown's grounding of postliberal politics in a set of "wounded attachments" (*States of Injury: Power and Freedom in Late Modernity* [Princeton University Press, 1995], chapter 5). See also Terry Eagleton, *The Ideology of the Aesthetic* (Oxford: Blackwell, 1991), 121; Grosz, *Volatile Bodies*; and Bakhtin, *Rabelais*.

28 The contrast could also be drawn with Kant, who insisted in *The Conflict of the Faculties* that a mature being should be able to rationally control their digestion (see Heather Merle Benbow, "Ways In, Ways Out: Theorizing the Kantian Body," *Body and Society* 9, no. 1 [2003]). For a defense of turning to Descartes instead of Kant, see Rorty, *Philosophy and the Mirror of Nature*.

29 "[T]he metaphorics of consuming, of sucking, of digesting structure the entire corpus of Hegel's texts just as much as the metaphorics of grasping and generating does," Werner Hamacher, *Pleroma: Reading in Hegel*, trans. N. Walker and S. Jarvis (London: Athlone Press, 1998), 234.

30 G.W. F. Hegel, *Philosophy of Nature*, trans. A. V. Miller (Oxford: Oxford University Press, 1970), 381–85.

31 Ibid., 395. For extensive discussions of this passage in *Philosophy of Nature*, see Mark C. E. Peterson, "Animals Eating Empiricists: Assimilation and Subjectivity

in Hegel's *Philosophy of Nature*," *The Owl of Minerva* 23, no. 1 (Fall 1991); and Tilottama Rajan, "(In)Digestible Material: Illness and Dialectic in Hegel's *The Philosophy of Nature*," in *Cultures of Taste/Theories of Appetite: Eating Romanticism*, ed. Timothy Morton (New York: Palgrave, 2004).

32 G. W. F. Hegel, *Science of Logic*, trans. A. V. Miller (Atlantic Highlands, N.J.: Humanities Press, 1969), 107.

33 G. W. F. Hegel, *Phenomenology of Spirit*, trans A. V. Miller (Oxford: Oxford University Press, 1977), 13.

34 Alexandre Kojève, *Introduction to the Reading of Hegel*, ed. Allan Bloom, trans. James H. Nichols (Ithaca: Cornell University Press, 1969), 4.

35 For example, see ibid., 17–18, 25.

36 This is an uneasy preference in Kojève, since at times he clearly admits that, through work, the world is humanized just as the human becomes worldly (ibid., 52–53). Ultimately, Kojève's imperialist tendencies seem to owe as much to his own brand of Marxist politics than to his otherwise quite digestive reading of Hegel.

37 While Hegel explicitly endorses a logic of contract, he warns against allowing the contract metaphor to bear too much political weight. It is, he argues, inappropriate to our most fundamental relations—marriage and citizenship—that consist of organic rather than mere legal bonds. See *The Philosophy of Right*, trans. T. M. Knox (Oxford: Oxford University Press, 1952), 58–59.

38 Rajan, "(In)Digestible Material."

39 Hegel, *Philosophy of Nature*, 405.

40 Ibid., 387 and compare with Descartes: "[Although] I have a body with which I am very closely united . . . it is certain that this 'I' . . . is entirely . . . distinct from my body" (*Meditations*, 132).

41 Hegel, *Phenomenology of Spirit*, 111–19.

42 Patchen Markell, *Bound by Recognition* (Princeton: Princeton University Press, 2003), 104.

43 Ibid.

44 Ibid., 22.

45 Ibid., 108.

46 Charles Taylor, "The Politics of Recognition," in *Multiculturalism*, ed. Amy Gutmann (Princeton: Princeton University Press 1994), 50.

47 Markell, *Bound by Recognition*, 36.

48 Grosz, *Volatile Bodies*, 193–94.

49 Markell, *Bound by Recognition*, 6.

50 Ibid., 12.

51 Ibid., 22.

52 Ibid., 104. We will return to this condition of shared vulnerability and its role in contemporary democratic theory in the Conclusion.

53 Marx, *Capital, Volume 1*, 342, 367.

54 Ibid., 198. Marx uses this term throughout the book.

55 Marx, *Capital, Volume 1*, 283, 290.

56 John Bellamy Foster, *Marx's Ecology: Materialism and Nature* (New York: Monthly Review Press, 2000).

57 Wendling, *Karl Marx on Technology and Alienation*, 62, 83–84.

58 Karl Marx, *Grundrisse*, trans. M Nicolaus (New York: Penguin, 1973), 85–100.

59 Marx, *Grundrisse*, 90–91.

60 See Gregory, *Scientific Materialism*; Rabinbach, *Human Motor*; Wendling, *Karl Marx on Technology and Alienation*.

61 Marx, *Capital, Volume 1*, 274–75.

62 Wendling *Karl Marx on Technology and Alienation*; Rabinbach, *Human Motor*, 45, 75–76.

63 Marx, *Capital, Volume 1*, 130.

64 Ibid., 126.

65 Marx, *Grundrisse*, 323.

66 Marx, *Capital, Volume 1*, 274.

67 Marx, *Grundrisse*, 90–94.

68 Ibid., 92.

69 Wendling, *Karl Marx on Technology and Alienation*, 82. Discussing a residual "mysticism" or "vitalism" at work in Marx's treatment of human labor-power, Wendling only gestures to this more conceptual violation of the first law of thermodynamics, chalking it up to an "ambivalence" on Marx's part about the creative power of human energies (ibid., 117–21).

70 Georg Lukács, *History and Class Consciousness*, trans. R. Livingstone (Cambridge: MIT Press, 1971), 83–110.

71 Marx, *Capital, Volume 1*, 163–77.The growing literature on commodity chains is entirely predicated on debunking this fetishism, tracing finished products to often-invisible forms of labor and exploitation. See Hughes and Reimer, *Geographies of Commodity Chains* or Pollan, *Omnivore's Dilemma*.

72 For more on how Marx reformulates agency and responsibility, see Lavin, *Politics of Responsibility*.

73 Nietzsche, *Genealogy of Morals*, 3.16.

74 Ibid., 2.1. "The German spirit is an indigestion: it does not finish with anything" (Nietzsche, *Ecce Homo*, 238).

75 Ibid., 2.11.

76 Ibid., 3.8.

77 Ibid., 2.2.

78 Ibid., 3.16.

79 Nietzsche, *Ecce Homo*, 215, 253.

80 Friedrich Nietzsche, *Thus Spoke Zarathustra*, trans. W. Kaufmann (New York: Vintage, 1966), section 4.

81 Melissa Orlie, "Impersonal Matter," in *New Materialisms: Ontology, Agency, and Politics*, ed. Diana Coole and Samantha Frost (Durham: Duke University Press, 2010).

82 Friedrich Nietzsche *Beyond Good and Evil*, trans. W. Kaufmann (New York: Vintage,

1966), part 6; Brian Leiter, *Routledge Philosophy Guidebook to Nietzsche on Morality* (New York: Routledge, 2002), 63–71.

83 Daniel Conway, *Nietzsche's Dangerous Game: Philosophy in the Twilight of the Idols (Modern European Philosophy)* (Oxford: Oxford University Press, 1997).

84 Nietzsche, *Genealogy of Morals*, 1.7.

85 Ibid., 1.6.

86 For a clear statement of this threat of nihilism, see Kass, *Hungry Soul.*

87 Orlie, "Impersonal Matter"; William Connolly, "Beyond Good and Evil: The Ethical Sensibility of Michel Foucault" *Political Theory* 21, no. 3 (1993); and Connolly, *Ethos of Pluralization.*

88 Orlie, "Impersonal Matter," 134.

89 "The excess of life over identity provides the fugitive source from which one comes to appreciate, and perhaps to love, the an-archy of being amidst the organ-ization of identity/difference" (Connolly, "Beyond Good and Evil," 371).

90 Connolly, "Beyond Good and Evil," 373.

91 Jay, *Downcast Eyes*; Weinek, "Digesting the Nineteenth Century."

92 Jay, *Downcast Eyes*, 338–52. Jay also posits that this explains why French aesthetics has always focused on painting whereas German aesthetics have tended toward music: the aesthetic pleasures of music do not depend on separation of subject and object but precisely on the collapse of that distance, as the sound enters the body and stimulates the ears (Jay, *Downcast Eyes*, 265).

93 See Gregory, *Scientific Materialism*; Mendelsohn, "Revolution and Reduction."

94 For another version of this argument, see Jonathan Havercroft, *Captives of Sovereignty* (Cambridge: Cambridge University Press, 2011).

95 See Jones, *Feast*; Glassner, *Gospel of Food.*

96 Warren Belasco's *Appetite for Change: How the Counterculture Took on the Food Industry* (New York: Pantheon Books, 1989) is the best example of this approach, linking an alternative diet to a spiritual reconciliation with the earth and a commitment to social justice. But see also Pollan, *Omnivore's Dilemma* and Kingsolver, *Animal, Vegetable, Miracle.*

97 See Pollan, "Our National Eating Disorder"; Glassner, *Gospel of Food.*

4. Responsibility and Disease in Obesity Politics

1 Sander Gilman, *Fat: A Cultural History of Obesity* (Cambridge: Polity Press, 2008), 30.

2 McDonald's denied that this decision had anything to do with the film.

3 According to its website, the CCF is "devoted to promoting personal responsibility and protecting consumer choices" and is "supported by restaurants, food companies and thousands of individual consumers" (http://www.consumerfreedom.com, accessed July 13, 2011). The website has a remarkable number of articles dedicated to criticizing Morgan Spurlock. *Super Size Me* has also inspired multiple

counterfilms with titles such as *Debunk the Junk*, *Portion-Size Me*, and *Fat Head* that seek to replicate Spurlock's experiment but with vastly different results.

4 Chuck Klosterman, "McDiculous," *Esquire*, May 1, 2004. In a corrective footnote, Klosterman offers that that election of George W. Bush is actually a slightly bigger problem.

5 In the film's opening voice-over, Spurlock asks, "Where does personal responsibility stop and corporate responsibility begin?" But after this, this terminology only appears twice, and both times are in pitches from a lawyer pursuing the now-prohibited lawsuits against fast food.

6 Stephen Shapin, "Eat and Run," *The New Yorker* January 16, 2006; see also Ellen Ruppel Shell, *The Hungry Gene: Inside the Story of the Obesity Industry* (New York: Grove Press 2002), 39; Stearns, *Fat History*, 249.

7 William Saletan, "Please Do Not Feed the Humans," *Slate*, September 2, 2006; Adam Drewnowski and S. E. Specter, "Poverty and Obesity: The Role of Energy Density and Energy Costs," *American Journal of Clinical Nutrition* 79 (2004).

8 Michael Gard and Jan Wright, *The Obesity Epidemic: Science, Morality, and Ideology* (New York: Routledge, 2005), 2.

9 Priscilla Wald, *Contagious: Cultures, Carriers, and the Outbreak Narrative* (Durham: Duke University Press, 2008).

10 Levenstein, *Paradox of Plenty*, 203.

11 Schwartz, *Never Satisfied*, chapter 6.

12 The Senate Nutrition Committee warned Americans about obesity in 1977, and the National Institutes of Heath (NIH) issued a report linking obesity to various diseases (e.g., hypertension, diabetes, and gout) in 1985. Covering this report for *Science*, Gina Kolata demonstrates the lack of clarity on the issue at this point, since her article is titled "Obesity Declared a Disease" (*Science* 227, no. 4690 [March 1985]), but the report itself does *not* actually declare obesity a disease, only that obesity causes these other diseases. Kolata's story concludes with the following statement from NIH panel chairman Jules Hirsch: "[T]here are multiple health hazards at . . . low levels of obesity. Obesity, therefore, is a disease." There will be more discussion of the definition of disease in the next section, but for now note that according to Hirsch's sloppy metric, working in a slaughterhouse, playing high school sports, and driving without a seatbelt could also be called diseases.

13 Critser, *Fat Land*.

14 Lebesco, *Revolting Bodies*; Anna Kirkland, *Fat Rights: Dilemmas of Difference and Personhood* (New York: NYU Press, 2008).

15 Gard and Wrigh, *Obesity Epidemic*; Gina Kolata, "For a World of Woes, We Blame Cookie Monsters," *New York Times*, October 29, 2006.

16 Mary Clare Jalonick, "Report Links School Lunches to National Security," Associated Press, April 20, 2010.

17 Lebesco, *Revolting Bodies*, 55.

18 "Overweight" is defined as a BMI over 25; "obese" is a BMI over 30. BMI has long been a controversial measure since its disregard of body type and muscle mass

mean that many extremely fit people have high BMIs. Still, BMI remains the gold standard in discourses of health and weight.

19 Marion Nestle, *Food Politics*, 11; Kelly Brownell, *Food Fight*, 10.

20 Paula Treichler, *How to Have Theory in an Epidemic: Cultural Chronicles of AIDS* (Durham: Duke University Press, 1999); Susan Sontag, *Illness as Metaphor and AIDS and Its Metaphors* (New York: Picador, 1990).

21 For example, Kim Chernin, *The Obsession: Reflections on the Tyranny of Slenderness* (New York: Harper Collins, 1981); and Susan Bordo, *Unbearable Weight*.

22 The Department of Health and Human Services officially classified obesity as a disease in 2004, though Medicare still does not cover most available treatments. Medicare does cover gastric bypass surgery in extreme cases.

23 Oliver explicitly indicts Nestle in this ploy, claiming that while she does not stand any immediate financial gain from the obesity epidemic, she uses it as "a useful weapon in the battle against corporate political influence" (*Fat Politics*, 48). Campos offers a similar critique of Critser, casting him as a victim of misguided white guilt instead of anticorporate activism (*Obesity Myth*, chapter 3).

24 Michael Pollan, "The Vegetable-Industrial Complex," *New York Times Magazine*, October 15, 2006; Critser, *Fat Land*, 126.

25 Oliver, *Fat Politics*, 12; Campos, *Obesity Myth*, 218.

26 Shell, *Obesity Industry*, 2; Glassner, *Gospel of Food*; Brian Wansink, *Mindless Eating: Why We Eat More than We Think* (New York: Bantam, 2010). Such claims are often overblown, ignoring the fact that "the food industry" comprises multiple, competing interests. The dairy industry, for example, suffers when the cola companies win access to school cafeterias. Nestle has made the most compelling argument for this term, however, when she claims that what allies each of these interests is an unstated commitment to avoid ever telling anybody to "eat less" of anything (*Food Politics*, 3).

27 Brillat-Savarin, *Physiology of Taste*, 245; Nidetch, *Story of Weight Watchers*, 14–15. See also Heyes, "Foucault Goes to Weight Watchers."

28 Judith Butler, *Precarious Life: The Powers of Mourning and Violence* (New York: Verso, 2004), chapter 1; and Butler *Giving an Account of Oneself*, chapter 3.

29 Brownell, *Food Fight*, 15. Shell's *The Hungry Gene* similarly notes the peculiarity of so much research attention being at the individual body despite copious evidence that we ought to be looking elsewhere.

30 Lebesco, *Revolting Bodies*, 21–23.

31 Brillat-Savarin, *Physiology of Taste*, 237.

32 Campos, *Obesity Myth*, chapter 3.

33 Critser, *Fat Land*, 49–53.

34 In a review of Critser's book, Pollan offers precisely this criticism: "[B]y the end of the book, the problem has largely, and somewhat inexplicably, been redefined in terms of personal responsibility" ("You Want Fries with That?" *The New York Times Book Review*, January 12, 2003).

35 See Esther Rothblum and Sondra Solovay, *The Fat Studies Reader* (New York: NYU Press, 2009).

36 Lebesco, *Revolting Bodies*, 49. On Lebesco's status in the fat acceptance movement, see Robin Wilson, "A 'Fat Studies' Scholar No Longer Fits the Picture," *Chronicle of Higher Education*, June 30, 2006.

37 Rothblum and Solovay's *Fat Studies Reader*, for example, opens with an "Invitation to Revolution" and closes with the "Fat Liberation Manifesto," the latter of which ends with "FAT PEOPLE OF THE WORLD, UNITE! YOU HAVE NOTHING TO LOSE." But both of these essays explain the aim of fat studies as the overweight finding acceptance by mainstream society. Valuable as this project might be, it surely falls squarely within the domain of liberal identity—rather than revolutionary—politics.

38 Schwartz, *Never Satisfied*, 213–21.

39 *Stedman's Medical Dictionary* defines disease as "an interruption, cessation, or disorder of body function, system, or organ." As Oliver points out, obesity does none of these things, though various *treatments for* obesity—most notably gastric bypass surgery—do all of them.

40 David Allison, Kevin Fontaine, JoAnn Manson, June Stevens, and Theodore VanItallie, "Annual Deaths Attributable to Obesity in the United States," *Journal of the American Medical Association* 282, no. 16 (1999).

41 A. H. Mokdad, J. S. Marks, D. F. Stroup, and J. L. Geberding, "Actual Causes of Death in the United States, 2000," *Journal of the American Medical Association* 291, no. 10 (2004).

42 Katherine Flegal, "Excess Deaths Associated with Underweight, Overweight, and Obesity," *Journal of the American Medical Association* 293, no. 15 (2005).

43 Oliver, *Fat Politics*, 41–2. The maps are available at http://www.cdc.gov/nccdphp/dnpa/obesity/trend/maps (accessed March 1, 2012).

44 Lavin and Russill, "The Ideology of the Epidemic"; Chris Russill, "Tipping Point Forewarnings of Climate Change: Some Implications of an Emerging Trend," *Environmental Communication* 2, no. 2 (July 2008); John Nguyet Erni, "Epidemic Imaginary: Performing Global Figurations of 'Third World AIDS,'" *Space and Culture* 9, no. 4 (November 2006).

45 The best selling of the relevant best sellers is Malcolm Gladwell's *The Tipping Point: How Little Things Can Make a Big Difference* (New York: Little, Brown, 2000). For a lengthier discussion of this trend and other contributions to the genre, see Lavin and Russill, "The Ideology of the Epidemic."

46 See Gilman, *Fat*, 23–43.

47 See Robin Marantz Henig, "Fat Factors," *New York Times Magazine*, August 13, 2006; or Gilman, *Fat*, 22–27.

48 See Shell, *The Hungry Gene*; Malcolm Gladwell, "The Pima Paradox," *The New Yorker*, February 2, 1998; or Christa Weil, "Heavy Questions," *New York Times Magazine*, January 2, 2005.

49 Nicholas Christakis and James Fowler, "The Spread of Obesity in a Large Social Network over 32 Years," *New England Journal of Medicine* 357, no. 4 (July 26, 2007).

50 Quoted in Gina Kolata "Study Says Obesity Can Be Contagious," *New York Times*,

July 25, 2007. Nicholas Christakis and James Fowler subsequently published "The Collective Dynamics of Smoking in a Large Social Network," *New England Journal of Medicine* 358, no. 21 (May 22, 2008), which makes exactly the same argument about smoking. They eventually parlayed this way of thinking into the popular best seller (from Gladwell's publisher) *Connected: The Surprising Power of Our Social Networks and How They Shape Our Lives* (New York: Little, Brown, 2009).

51 See Bordo, *Unbearable Weight*, 66–69.

52 See Gilman, *Fat*, chapter 4.

53 As Oliver puts this, "the reason that so many people think the rise of obesity is cause for alarm is because of our own chronic feelings of helplessness" (*Fat Politics*, 77).

54 Nikolas Rose, *Politics of Life Itself: Biomedicine, Power, and Subjectivity in the Twenty-First Century* (Princeton: Princeton University Press, 2006).

55 Nancy Lofholm, "Heavy Infant in Grand Junction Denied Health Insurance," *Denver Post*, October 10, 2009.

56 Kirsten Ostherr, *Cinematic Prophylaxis: Globalization and Contagion in the Discourse of World Health* (Durham: Duke University Press, 2005).

57 Foucault, *Society Must Be Defended*, 255.

58 Jean-François Lyotard, *The Postmodern Condition: A Report on Knowledge*, trans. B. Massumi (Minneapolis: University of Minnesota Press, 1984); Latour, *Politics of Nature*; Hardt and Negri, *Empire*, *Multitude*, and *Commonwealth*

59 Pollan, *Omnivore's Dilemma*, 257.

60 William Connolly, *IdentityDifference: Democratic Negotiations of Political Paradox* (Ithaca: Cornell University Press, 1991), 19–27.

61 See Gladwell, "Pima Paradox."

62 Taubes, *Good Calories*, xix.

63 Ibid., 91.

64 Pollan, *Omnivore's Dilemma*.

65 Pollan, *Food Rules*.

66 Glassner, *Gospel of Food*.

67 Foucault, *Birth of Biopolitics*. Foucault was not entirely consistent with regard to the presumed relationship between the paradigm of sovereignty and that of biopolitics, at times suggesting that the latter would supplant the former and at other times explaining how these two paradigms worked in tandem in modern liberalism. See Thomas Lemke, *Biopolitics: An Advanced Introduction*, trans. Eric Frederick Trump (New York: NYU Press, 2011). My argument here allies with the latter interpretation, in which biopolitical rule supplements—rather than supplants—sovereignty.

68 Fredric Jameson, "Cognitive Mapping," in *Marxism and the Interpretation of Culture*, ed. C. Nelson and L. Grossberg (Urbana: University of Illinois Press, 1985).

5. The Year of Eating Politically

1 Berry, *What are People For?*, 145.

2 Murray Bookchin, *The Modern Crisis* (Cheektowaga, N.Y.: Black Rose Books, 1987).

3 Julie Guthman, *Agrarian Dreams: The Paradox of Organic Farming in California* (Berkeley: University of California Press, 2004).

4 Samuel Fromartz, *Organic, Inc.: Natural Foods and How They Grew* (New York: Harcourt, 2006), ix.

5 Levenstein, *Paradox of Plenty*, 183.

6 On the difficulties encountered in developing "ethnic" (i.e., Mexican, Italian, and Chinese) chain restaurants in the United States, see Glassner, *Gospel of Food*, chapter 5.

7 Belasco, *Appetite for Change*, 49–50.

8 Nor—given how much agricultural technology can be traced to military research—is it entirely a coincidence that the man who won a 1920 Nobel Prize for developing synthetic fertilizer, Fritz Haber, also developed Zyklon B, the gas used in Hitler's concentration camps (Pollan, *Omnivore's Dilemma*, 43).

9 Laura Shapiro, "Suddenly, It's a Panic for Organic," *Newsweek*, March 1989.

10 For more detailed versions of this story, see Belasco *Appetite for Change*; Fromartz, *Organic, Inc.*; Guthman, *Agrarian Dreams*; Levenstein, *Paradox of Plenty*; or Pollan, *Omnivore's Dilemma*.

11 Kingsolver, *Animal, Vegetable, Miracle*; Bill McKibben, *Deep Economy: The Wealth of Communities and the Durable Future* (New York: Times Books, 2007); Alisa Smith and J. B. MacKinnon, *Plenty: One Man, One Woman, and a Raucous Year of Eating Locally* (New York: Harmony Books, 2007); Adam Gopnik, "Annals of Agriculture—New York Local: Eating the Fruits of the Five Burroughs," *The New Yorker*, September 3, 2007. Contributions to the genre continue to proliferate. See Betty Fussell, *Raising Steaks: The Life and Times of American Beef* (New York: Houghton Mifflin, 2008); Steven Rinella, *American Buffalo: In Search of a Lost Icon* (New York: Spiegel & Grau, 2008); and Novella Carpenter, *Farm City: The Education of an Urban Farmer* (New York: Penguin, 2009).

12 John Cloud, "Eating Better than Organic," *Time*, March 2, 2007.

13 I have not mentioned a competing trend, *Slow Food*, in part because despite casual appropriations this term actually refers to a specific organization, and in part because the concern with slowness seems but one manifestation of a concern with locality. In their monograph *Slow Living*, Wendy Parkins and Geoffrey Craig explicitly cast time and space as coequal concerns, alongside pleasure (Wendy Parkins and Geoffrey Craig, *Slow Living* [New York: Berg 2006]). For more on concerns about speed owing to a postmodern collapse of space, see Harvey, *Condition of Postmodernity*.

14 Bill McKibben, *The End of Nature* (New York: Random House, 1989).

15 Bill McKibben, *Enough: Staying Human in an Engineered Age* (New York: Henry Holt, 2003).

16 McKibben, *Deep Economy*, 65; Pollan, *Omnivore's Dilemma*, 167.

17 For an even clearer example, see Richard Manning's essay "The Oil We Eat," *Harper's*, February 2004.

18 Cullather shows how this thermodynamic thinking has directed U.S. foreign policy since the early twentieth century, especially as it cast global hunger as a "caloric deficit," a measure that "can be tabulated as easily as currency or petroleum" ("Foreign Policy of the Calorie").

19 James McWilliams, *Just Food: Where Locavores Get It Wrong and How We Can Truly Eat Responsibly* (New York: Little, Brown, 2009).

20 Parkins and Craig, *Slow Living*, 62.

21 I discussed this issue in chapter 1. For a sampling of people making this argument, see Henri Lefebvre, *The Production of Space*, trans. D. Nicholson-Smith (Oxford: Blackwell 1991); Bordo, *Flight to Objectivity*; Harvey, *Condition of Postmodernity*; Brown, *Walled States*.

22 Brian Halweil, *Eat Here: Reclaiming Homegrown Pleasures in a Global Supermarket* (New York: Norton, 2004), 10, 16.

23 McKibben, *Deep Economy*, 109.

24 Bulliet, *Hunters, Herders, and Hamburgers*, 3.

25 Pollan, *Omnivore's Dilemma*, chapter 9.

26 See also Brown, *States of Injury*, 69.

27 Kingsolver, *Animal, Vegetable, Miracle*, 23.

28 Cohen, *Consumer's Republic*, 228.

29 Peter Singer and Jim Mason, *The Way We Eat: Why Our Food Choices Matter* (New York: Rodale, 2006).

30 Gopnik, "New York Local."

31 Kingsolver, *Animal, Vegetable, Miracle*, 7–8.

32 Kingsolver, *Animal, Vegetable, Miracle*, 2.

33 Pollan, *Omnivore's Dilemma*, 245.

34 Smith and MacKinnon, *Plenty*, 71–3. For another critique of localist elitism, see Glassner's "fast food populism" that celebrates the convenient and affordable foods that locavores malign but on which most city dwellers depend (*Gospel of Food*, chapter 6).

35 Kingsolver, *Animal, Vegetable, Miracle*, 153.

36 Ibid., 307.

37 Ibid., 249.

38 See Carlo Petrini, *Slow Food Nation: Why Our Food Should Be Good, Clean, and Fair*, trans. C. Furlan and J. Hunt (New York: Rizzoli Ex Libris, 2007); Parkins and Craig, *Slow Living*; or Corby Kummer, *The Pleasures of Slow Food* (San Francisco: Chronicle Books, 2002), which are all much more clear about the movement's roots in radical left politics.

39 Halweil, *Eat Here*, 157–58.

40 Ibid., 165.

41 Even McWilliams, at the end of his critique of locavorism, offers a baffling conflation of citizenship and consumerism: "Our job *as consumers* is not what it used to be. It is, in essence, less to make choices among the current range of food options,

and more to advocate for changes that would help develop a sound twenty-first-century food system, one in which our collective choices might matter" (*Just Food*, 213–14, emphasis added). The changes he proceeds to recommend are entirely technological.

42 Fromartz frames his book on organics as an issue of trust (*Organic, Inc.*, ix), and Levenstein notes how the organics movement coincides with a proliferation of "alternative" medicines, signaling a similar lack of confidence in the American medical establishment (*Paradox of Plenty*, chapter 13).

43 Fromartz, *Organic, Inc.*, chapter 6; Pollan, *Omnivore's Dilemma*, 155–56.

44 Whole Foods founder and (until 2009) CEO John Mackey is an avowed libertarian, and the chain is known for championing the benevolent labor practices designed to frustrate unions.

45 Guthman, *Agrarian Dreams*, 12, 14.

46 Halweil, *Eat Here*, chapter 9. The most common personality here is Joel Salatin, owner/operator of Polyface Farms and self-described "Christian-conservative-libertarian-environmentalist-lunatic farmer" (Pollan, *Omnivore's Dilemma*, 125). A more striking character, however, is probably Arthur Harvey, an organic blueberry farmer who sued the USDA in 2002 and who (again evoking Thoreau) has refused to pay federal income taxes since 1959 due to his opposition to military spending (Fromartz, *Organic, Inc.*, introduction). Such heroic individuals are a staple of the literature.

47 Pollan, *Omnivore's Dilemma*, 257.

48 For a more specific critique of Pollan's politics and his relationship to neoliberalism, see my "Pollanated Politics, or, the Neoliberal's Dilemma" (*Politics and Culture* 2 [April 2009]).

49 Bookchin, *Modern Crisis*, 90; see also J. K. Gibson-Graham, *A Postcapitalist Politics* (Minneapolis: University of Minnesota Press, 2006), chapter 4.

50 Smith and MacKinnon, *Plenty*, 173.

51 Pollan celebrates Salatin for farming in a manner that his land "will be in no way diminished by the process—in fact, it will be the better for it, lusher, more fertile, even springier underfoot," casting the farmer as the quintessential Lockean subject, adding value to the land by cultivating it (*Omnivore's Dilemma*, 127).

52 Guthman, *Agrarian Dreams*, 175.

53 Fromartz, *Organic, Inc.*, chapter 2.

54 See Marx, *Grundrisse*, 85–100 and *Capital, Volume 1*, 198. Or see chapter 2.

55 Petrini, *Slow Food Nation*, 129–35.

56 Cohen, *Consumer's Republic*, 404–5.

57 Jodi Dean, *Democracy and Other Neoliberal Fantasies* (Durham: Duke University Press, 2009); Timothy W. Luke, *Ecocritique: Contesting the Politics of Nature, Economy, and Culture* (Minneapolis: University of Minnesota Press, 1997).

58 Luke, *Ecocritique*, 119.

59 Dean, *Democracy and Other Neoliberal Fantasies*, 33.

60 Pollan, *Omnivore's Dilemma*, 257.

61 Pollan, "You Are What You Grow," in *Manifestos on the Future of Food and Seed*, ed. V. Shiva (South End Press, 2007), 139.

62 See Michael Pollan, "Weed It and Reap," *New York Times*, November 4, 2007; Imhoff, *Food Fight*; and Pollan's foreword to Imhoff, "Don't Call It the 'Farm Bill,' Call It the 'Food Bill.'"

63 Guthman, *Agrarian Dreams*, 184–85.

64 Brown, *States of Injury*, 98.

6. The Meat We Don't Eat

1 Rebecca Ruiz, "Are You Eating Too Much Meat?" *Forbes*, 24 March 2009, accessed February 12, 2012, http://www.forbes.com/2009/03/24/eating-red-meat-lifestyle-health-red-meat-study.html.

2 J. M. Coetzee, *The Lives of Animals* (Princeton: Princeton University Press, 1999), 69.

3 Peter Dauvergne, *The Shadows of Consumption: Consequences for the Global Environment* (Cambridge: MIT Press, 2008), chapter 18.

4 Peter Singer, *Practical Ethics*, 2nd ed. (Cambridge: Cambridge University Press, 1993).

5 Or do they? In an opinion piece titled "We Eat Horses, Don't We?" (*New York Times*, March 5, 2007), Christa Weil argues that Americans have not infrequently resorted to eating horse when beef is in short supply, most recently in the 1970s. Further, the difference between drinking blood and receiving a blood transfusion, between eating human flesh and receiving an organ transplant, remains open for debate.

6 Thanks to Jodi Dean for noting this.

7 Steven Shaviro, *The Cinematic Body* (Minneapolis: University of Minnesota Press, 1993), 84.

8 Joseph Valente, *Dracula's Crypt: Bram Stoker, Irishness, and the Question of Blood* (Urbana: University of Illinois Press, 2002).

9 Marx, *Capital, Volume 1*, 342.

10 George Fitzhugh, *Cannibals All! Or Slaves Without Masters* (Cambridge: Belknap Press, 1988).

11 Frank Lestringant, *Cannibals: The Discovery and Representation of the Cannibal from Columbus to Jules Verne* (Berkeley: University of California Press, 1997), 15.

12 Steven Lukes, *Liberals and Cannibals: The Implications of Diversity* (New York: Verso, 2003), 30.

13 Michel de Montaigne, "Of Cannibals," in *The Complete Works: Essays, Travel Journal, Letters*, trans. D. Frame (New York: Knopf, 2003); and Jonathan Swift, *A Modest Proposal and Other Writings*, ed. C. Fabricante (New York: Penguin, 2009).

14 Kass, *Hungry Soul*, 99, 109.

15 W. Arens, *The Man-Eating Myth: Anthropology and Anthropophagy* (Oxford: Oxford University Press, 1979), 16. Taking a page from Montaigne, Arens also tries to invert the narrative by claiming that Tanzanian natives often suspect Europeans

of drinking human blood—a suspicion that Arens cheekily links to an attempt by the British to mount a blood drive there during World War II (12–13).

16 Lestringent, *Cannibals*, 7, 6.

17 Claude Rawson, "The Horror, the Holy Horror," *Times Literary Supplement*, October 31, 1997.

18 Jared Diamond, *Collapse: How Societies Choose to Fail or Succeed* (New York: Viking, 2005).

19 Rawson, "The Horror, the Holy Horror."

20 Nietzsche, *Genealogy of Morals*, 3.17.

21 Charles Stahler, "How Many Adults Are Vegetarian?" *Vegetarian Journal* 4 (2006). The numbers are difficult to verify in part because there is substantial disagreement about what counts as a vegetarian (eaters of eggs, gelatin, rennet, fish, etc.?), and in part because, as any practicing vegetarian can attest, it is not at all uncommon for people to claim to be vegetarian one day but not the next.

22 United States Department of Agriculture, *Agriculture Fact Book, 2001–2002* and *Agricultural Statistics 2007* (Washington, D.C.: United States Government Printing Office, 2002 and 2007). "Meat" here refers to beef, veal, lamb, pork, poultry, and fish.

23 John Robbins's *Diet for a New America* (Walpole, N.H.: Stillpoint, 1987), for instance, perhaps the book most well known for focusing on the medical evidence for the benefits of a vegetarian diet, opens with a "dream of a society at peace with its conscience because it respects and lives in harmony with all life forms" (xiii) and is divided into three sections of roughly equal length: ethics, nutrition, and environment.

24 Tom Regan, *The Case for Animal Rights* (Berkeley: University of California Press, 2004); Peter Singer, *Animal Liberation* (New York: Harper Collins, 1975) and *Practical Ethics*; Carol Adams, *The Sexual Politics of Meat: A Feminist-Vegetarian Critical Theory* (New York: Continuum, 2000) and *Neither Beast nor Man: Feminism and the Defense of Animals* (New York: Continuum, 1994).

25 Kass, *Hungry Soul*, 2–5.

26 Ibid., 99, 110, 117.

27 Leon Kass, "The Wisdom of Repugnance," *The New Republic* 216, no. 22 (June 2, 1997).

28 Steven Shapin, "Vegetable Love," *The New Yorker*, January 22, 2007.

29 J. M. Coetzee, *Elizabeth Costello* (New York: Penguin, 2003) and *Lives of Animals*; Jennifer Schuessler, "Mau-Mauing the Flesh Eaters," *New York Times*, November 13, 2009.

30 Jonathan Safran Foer, *Eating Animals* (Boston: Little, Brown, 2009), 264.

31 Jennifer Howard, "Creature Consciousness," *Chronicle of Higher Education*, October 18, 2009.

32 Jacques Derrida, *The Animal That Therefore I Am*, trans. D. Wills (New York: Fordham University Press, 2008); Donna Haraway, *The Companion Species Manifesto: Dogs, People, and Significant Otherness* (Chicago: Prickly Paradigm Press, 2003); and *When Species Meet* (Minneapolis: University of Minnesota Press, 2008); Cary

Wolfe, *Animal Rites: American Culture, the Discourse of Species, and Posthumanist Theory* (Chicago: University of Chicago Press, 2003) and *What Is Posthumanism?* (Minneapolis: University of Minnesota Press, 2010).

33 Derrida, *The Animal That Therefore I Am*; Wolfe, *Animal Rites*, 7.

34 Wolfe, *What Is Posthumanism?*, xv.

35 Tristram Stuart, *The Bloodless Revolution: A Cultural History of Vegetarianism from 1600 to Modern Times* (New York: W. W. Norton & Company, 2006), xvii–xx.

36 This periodization overlaps with Harriet Ritvo's *The Animal Estate: The English and Other Creatures in the Victorian Age* (Cambridge: Harvard University Press, 1987), which identifies a similar ambivalence about the manipulation of animals consequent to the development of veterinary science in the nineteenth century.

37 John Berger, *About Looking* (New York: Random House, 1980); Bulliet, *Hunters, Herders, and Hamburgers*.

38 Pollan, *Omnivore's Dilemma*, 306.

39 Mitchell continues, "Resistance, because acknowledging the claim that animals might have or deserve rights entails a revolution in thinking and behavior so profound that it would shake the foundations of human society. Anxiety because we suspect there is something compelling and irresistible about the concept of animal rights, at least insofar as we are all dimly aware that human life as now constituted is based on the mass slaughter of billions of animals accompanied by untold suffering" (in Wolfe, *Animal Rites*, ix).

40 This is obviously the case with the footage in "Meet Your Meat," the infamous video from People for the Ethical Treatment of Animals (PETA), which portrays such mistreatment of animals that viewers might be reacting less to the slaughter than to the sheer cruelty. But I have had very similar results showing footage of very careful and heavily regulated slaughter, such as that in the Austrian film *Unser Täglich Brot* (*Our Daily Bread*) directed by Nikolaus Geyrhalter (Nikolaus Geyrhalter Filmproduktion, 2005), which could not possibly be charged with sensationalism or sentimentality.

41 The term comes from Jon Mooallem, "Carnivores, Capitalists, and the Meat We Read," *Believer*, October 2005. For more on the concept, see Chad Lavin, "Factory Farms in a Consumer Society," *American Studies* 50, no. 1/2 (Spring/Summer 2009).

42 Pollan, *Omnivore's Dilemma*, 231. Though Pollan initially mocks "the whole macho conceit that the most authentic encounter with nature is one that comes through the sight of a gun and ends with a large mammal dead on the ground" (*Omnivore's Dilemma*, 336), he reluctantly admits after his kill that manly men like Ernest Hemingway were on to something.

43 Haraway, *When Species Meet*, 295–99.

44 Steven Rinella, *The Scavenger's Guide to Haute Cuisine* (New York: Miramax Books, 2006) and *American Buffalo*; Elizabeth Kolbert, "Flesh of Your Flesh," *The New Yorker*, November 9, 2009; Peggy Orenstein, "The Femivore's Dilemma," *New York Times Magazine*, March 11, 2010.

45 Kurt Soller, "Head to Hoof," *Newsweek*, January 28, 2009; Betty Fussell, "Earning

Her Food," *New York Times Magazine*, March 22, 2010. For a critique of these full-throated celebrations of killing animals, see B. R. Myers, "The Moral Crusade against Foodies," *Atlantic*, March 2011.

46 Michael Schaffer, *One Nation Under Dog: Adventures in the New World of Prozac-Popping Puppies, Dog-Park Politics, and Organic Pet Food* (New York: Henry Holt, 2009).

47 Haraway, *When Species Meet*, 205–6. Such cases bleed into ongoing debates about the increasing reliance on service animals and informs ongoing controversies stemming from people taking birds, monkeys, and even horses into various public places to deal with medical conditions ranging from diabetes to schizophrenia. See Rebecca Skloot, "Creature Comforts," *New York Times Magazine* (December 31, 2008). Full disclosure: the author currently lives with nonhuman animals named Lola, Levon, and Francis (though he did not pick those names, and he has never taken any of them to work).

48 Marjorie Garber, *Dog Love* (New York: Touchstone Books, 1996), 32.

49 Marc Fellenz, *The Moral Menagerie: Philosophy and Animal Rights* (Urbana: University of Illinois Press, 2007), 20.

50 Kass, *Hungry Soul*, 5, 110.

51 Donna Haraway, "A Cyborg Manifesto," in *Simians, Cyborgs, and Women* (New York: Routledge, 1991), 151–52; and *When Species Meet*, 3.

52 Wolfe, *Animal Rites*, 17.

53 Foer, *Eating Animals*, 24–29. This proposal, along with a recipe for a stewed dog, was printed in the *Wall Street Journal* as "Let Them Eat Dog," December 31, 2008.

54 While Haraway defines "companion species" as a coevolutionary relationship between humans and nonhumans, it is anything but clear why the human relation with cows would be any less central to her analysis than our relationship with dogs. In the "coevolutionary bargain" struck between corn and humans that is the focus of Pollan's books, it is clear that propagating and eating are essential aspects of what Haraway calls "biosociality." It is unclear, that is, what allows her to claim that "generally speaking, one does not eat one's companion animals" (Haraway, *Companion Species Manifesto*, 14), or what—aside from an oddly parochial notion of cohabitation—justifies her claim that dogs are companion species but cows are not.

55 Haraway, *When Species Meet*, chapter 10.

56 Ibid., 295.

57 Ibid., 297.

58 Ibid., 293.

59 Ibid., 293–94.

60 Ibid., 295.

61 Jane Bennett, *Vibrant Matter: A Political Ecology of Things* (Durham: Duke University Press, 2010), xi; Stephen White, *The Ethos of a Late-Modern Citizen* (Cambridge: Harvard University Press, 2009), 97; Jacques Rancière, *Dissensus: On Politics and Aesthetics*, trans. S. Corcoran (New York: Continuum, 2010), chapter 13.

62 See, for example, Dean, *Democracy and Other Neoliberal Fantasies*.

63 Bennett, *Vibrant Matter*, xii.

64 Singer, *Animal Liberation*, 162.

65 Singer's involvement in the Great Ape Project (which seeks to confer legal rights on chimpanzee, gorillas, and other nonhuman apes) and his endorsement of California's Proposition 2 (which effectively prohibits many conventional forms of raising livestock starting in 2015) would be notable exceptions from this claim. Thanks to Larry Torcello for reminding me of these positions.

66 Haraway, *When Species Meet*, 295.

67 Regan, *Case for Animal Rights*, 353.

68 Foer, *Eating Animals*, 266.

69 Though she never advocates vegetarianism, Bennett does promote an ethical approach to human/nonhuman relations that stems from "a shared experience of harm" (*Vibrant Matter*, 100). Given the realities of industrial meat production, however, it seems disingenuous at best to suggest that humans and nonhumans have an even remotely similar (or shared) experience of harm. More harshly, we might say that this *ethical* approach to nonhumans is blind to interspecies *politics*.

70 Both Stuart and Foer end their books with discussions of the political implications of vegetarianism, and for both those implications are found in environmentalism.

71 Wolfe, *What Is Posthumanism?*, 47.

72 Wolfe, *Animal Rites*, 7, 207.

73 See Wolin, *Politics and Vision*.

74 Latour, *Politics of Nature*, 6, 22.

75 Bennett, *Vibrant Matter*, 31, 115, 119. Bennett more often opts for the term "assemblage" over "network," though her work is clearly attempting to develop a political sensibility appropriate to a network society, and it does this in part through a consideration of digestion.

76 Ibid., 122.

77 Ibid., 121.

78 Wolfe, *Animal Rites*, 36.

79 Judith Butler, "Contingent Foundations," in *Feminist Contentions: A Philosophical Exchange*, ed. Seyla Benhabib, Judith Butler, Drucilla Cornell, and Nancy Fraser (New York: Routledge, 1995), 36.

Conclusion

1 In *Why Americans Hate Politics* (New York: Simon & Schuster, 1992), E. J. Dionne pointed to polarization, corruption, and cynicism. In claiming that we are *disgusted* by politics, however, I mean to say that it is not just a corruption of the process—but the very process itself—that is unpleasant.

2 Nietzsche, *Genealogy of Morals*, 2.7. Though the "*different* kind of spirit" that Nietzsche summons—one that is "strengthened by war and victory, for whom conquest, adventure, danger, and even pain have become needs" (Nietzsche, *Genealogy of Morals*, 2.24)—is difficult to read as a *democratic* spirit, it is the kind

of *vulnerable* and *engaged* spirit (prepared to be wounded and violated) that is essential to a democratic ethos. More on this later.

3 Miller, *The Anatomy of Disgust*. Other contributions, most of which will be discussed later in the chapter, include Martha Nussbaum's *Hiding from Humanity: Disgust, Shame, and the Law* (Princeton University Press, 2004); Winfried Menninghaus's *Disgust: The Theory and History of a Strong Sensation*, trans. H. Eiland and J. Golb (Albany: SUNY Press, 2003); a recent translation of Aurel Kolnai's *On Disgust*, ed. with an introduction by B. Smith and C. Korsmeyer (Peru, Ill.: Open Court Press, 2003); Julia Kristeva's *Powers of Horror: An Essay on Abjection*, trans. L. Roudiez (New York: Columbia University Press, 1982); Rachel Herz's popular *That's Disgusting: Unraveling the Mysteries of Repulsion* (New York: W. W. Norton & Company, 2012); and Leon Kass's "The Wisdom of Repugnance."

4 Miller, *The Anatomy of Disgust*, 10.

5 Ibid., 2.

6 Ibid., 163–70. Miller draws directly from the curious *Oxford English Dictionary* (second edition) entry for disgust: "This and all the cognate words appear after 1600. They are not used by Shakespeare."

7 For example, Paul Rozin, "Food Is Fundamental, Fun, Frightening, and Far-reaching," *Social Research* 66, no. 1 (Winter 1999); Paul Rozin and April Fallon, "A Perspective on Disgust," *Psychological Review* 94, no. 1 (1987).

8 Miller, *The Anatomy of Disgust*, 6.

9 Ibid., 50. Returning to the argument from chapter 6, we might suggest that cannibalism is disgusting because it is both human and nonhuman simultaneously: the cannibal is inhuman for rejecting the codes that (supposedly) distinguish us from animals, but if the cannibal is not human, it cannot be a cannibal.

10 Miller, *The Anatomy of Disgust*, 97.

11 For Miller, Douglas's work, which is not about disgust exactly but about dirt and taboo, is too structural and is thus unable to explain why feces might remain disgusting even if it is not *out of place* (e.g., when it is in the toilet). Defecating in a toilet, after all, does not violate any system at all, but is precisely following the system: food goes in, gets digested, and the unused portion is expelled into its designated receptacle. But Miller speculates this may be why vomit is more disgusting than feces: "Only feces is playing by the rules" (*The Anatomy of Disgust*, 96).

12 William Connolly, *Why I Am Not a Secularist* (Minneapolis: University of Minnesota Press, 1999), 163.

13 Miller, *The Anatomy of Disgust*, 97.

14 Sigmund Freud, "Negation" in *The Freud Reader*, ed. Peter Gay (New York: W. W. Norton and Company, 1995), 668.

15 Kristeva, *Powers of Horror*, 2.

16 Ibid., 37.

17 Miller, *The Anatomy of Disgust*, 50–58.

18 Nietzsche, *Genealogy of Morals*, 2.11.

19 Invoking the concept—but not the term—of a fetish, Pollan argues that consuming

industrial meat requires "an almost heroic act of not knowing or, now, forgetting" (*Omnivore's Dilemma*, 84).

20 Nussbaum, *Hiding from Humanity* 88.

21 Ibid., 16–17.

22 Ibid., 93.

23 For example, Wolin, *Politics and Vision*; Brown, *States of Injury*; Grosz, *Volatile Bodies*, 193–94.

24 Nussbaum, *Hiding from Humanity*, 92.

25 Lebesco, *Revolting Bodies*, 1.

26 Anna Kirkland, *Fat Rights*.

27 Lebesco, *Revolting Bodies*, 56; Paul Ernsberger, "Does Social Class Explain the Connection Between Weight and Health?" in *The Fat Studies Reader*, ed. Rothblum and Solovay (New York: NYU Press, 2009). Jerry Mosher argues that men in U.S. situation comedies grew increasingly fat as "a televisual symbol of downward mobility" ("Setting Free the Bears: Refiguring Fat Men on Television," in *Bodies Out of Bounds: Fatness and Transgression*, ed. Jana Evans Braziel and Kathleen Lebesco [Berkeley: University of California Press, 2001], 168). In particular, patriarchs on such shows as *All in the Family*, *The Honeymooners*, and *Roseanne*, embody "the growing alienation of white men in general. . . . In [Archie] Bunker's paunch . . . fat was established as a televisual symbol of white heterosexual masculinity losing its definition, rendered soft and impotent" (ibid., 169).

28 Lebesco, *Revolting Bodies*, 56.

29 See Mary Midgley, "Biotechnology and Monstrosity: Why We Should Pay Attention to the 'Yuk Factor,'" *Hastings Center Report* 30, no. 5 (September–October, 2000); Charles Schmidt, "The Yuck Factor: When Disgust Meets Discovery," *Environmental Health Perspectives* 116, no. 12 (December 2008); Koerner, "Will Lab-Grown Meat Save the Planet."

30 Mary Midgley, "Biotechnology and Monstrosity," 9, emphasis added. This is only one (and probably not the dominant) critical reaction to GMOs. Most activists, it has been noted, tend to invoke the economic (rather than genetic) consequences of biotechnology; their concern surrounds the ownership of seeds and other vital resource rather that the perversion of nature. See McWilliams, *Just Food*; or Rachel Schurman and William Munro, *Fighting for the Future of Food: Activists versus Agribusiness in the Struggle over Biotechnology* (Minneapolis: University of Minnesota Press, 2010). Indeed, even ecofeminists like Vandana Shiva rarely resort to the rhetoric of disgust when criticizing genetic modification of plants and animals, even as they invoke a romantic and troublesome ideal of species purity. See Shiva, *Stolen Harvest: The Hijacking of the Global Food Supply* (Boston: South End Press, 2000), 32. Nevertheless, as the Midgely quote suggests, this particular attack on GMOs is quite analogous to the debates about meat in chapter 6.

31 Kass does not use the word *disgust* in the essay, though he uses words like offensive, grotesque, revolting, repugnant, repellent, and repulsive somewhat interchangeably, suggesting that he is talking about the same thing.

32 Kass, *Hungry Soul*, 146.

33 Ibid., 148. To be sure, the fact that Americans *do* freely eat ice cream cones in public is, for Kass, indicative of "[m]odern America's rising tide of informality [that] has already washed out many long-standing customs . . . that served well to regulate the boundary between public and private" and that did not compel others "to witness our shameful behavior" (Kass, *Hungry Soul*, 149). For Kass, this "rising tide" is destroying our nation's moral fabric.

34 Ibid., 149.

35 Ibid., 152.

36 Ibid., 158–9.

37 Kass, "Wisdom of Repugnance."

38 Nussbaum, *Hiding from Humanity*, 14. This parallels Markell's claim that the politics of recognition is built on "a misrecognition of the basic conditions of human activity" (*Bound by Recognition*, 22). See chapter 3.

39 Nussbaum, *Hiding from Humanity*, 13. Connolly makes much the same point in his reflection on nose-picking; disgust, he declares, "sometimes breeds ethical thoughtlessness" (*Why I Am Not a Secularist*, 163).

40 Nussbaum, *Hiding from Humanity* 102.

41 Roberto Esposito, *Bios: Biopolitics and Philosophy*, trans. T. Campbell (Minneapolis: University of Minnesota Press, 2008) and *Communitas*; Judith Butler, *Frames of War: When Is Life Grievable?* (New York: Verso, 2009) and *Precarious Life*.

42 Esposito, *Communitas*, 12. See also Lefort, *Political Forms of Modern Society*, 298–303; Lemke, *Biopolitics*, 9–15.

43 Esposito, *Communitas*, 14.

44 Again, Warner, in *Publics and Counterpublics*, suggests a similar explanation for the politics of tolerance and homosexuality. As evidenced by policies like Don't Ask Don't Tell and the popular refrain that nobody cares "what you do in your own bedroom," it is not homosexuality *as such* but homosexuality *in public* that offends.

45 Esposito, *Communitas*, 7–14.

46 Butler, *Precarious Life*, 23.

47 Ibid., xiii. In using our vulnerability—our ability to suffer—rather than our capacities for speech, rationality, or agency to anchor a commitment to democracy, this argument demonstrates an unlikely affinity with the (liberal) vegetarian theory discussed in the previous chapter. Normatively, this allows Butler to take roughly the same position as Frost in *Lessons from a Materialist Thinker*. What is peculiar about Frost's argument, as I argued earlier, is that she claims to find this commitment to community in Hobbes.

48 Miller, *The Anatomy of Disgust*, 50.

49 Nussbaum, *Hiding from Humanity*, 17.

50 It is worth noting that whereas Butler invokes this vulnerability to invoke the possibility of a generous and democratic global community, Nussbaum voices its value through the language of tolerance. For more on the inadequacies of such an appeal to tolerance, especially as it, like other ethical modes of reasoning, "substitutes emotional and personal vocabularies for political ones," see Wendy

Brown, *Regulating Aversion: Tolerance in the Age of Identity and Empire* (Princeton: Princeton University Press, 2006), 16. This critique suggests that Nussbaum's approach participates in the apolitical logic of the ethical turn discussed in the previous chapter.

51 Pollan, *Omnivore's Dilemma*, 255.

52 For example, Glassner, *Gospel of Food*; Pollan, "Our National Eating Disorder."

53 Latour, *Politics of Nature*, 22.

54 Butler, *Precarious Life*, xiii.

55 Haraway, *When Species Meet*, 295.

56 Bennett, *Vibrant Matter*, 104.

57 Pollan, *Omnivore's Dilemma*, 257. Pollan is far from alone here; this empowering note is a staple of the literature. Even Schlosser, after he admits that Congress is unlikely to adopt any of the urgent reforms he recommends because our representatives are completely in the pocket of big corporations, ends his book with a declaration of individual empowerment through consumerism: "Even in this fast food nation, you can still have it your way" (270).

58 Ibid., 257.

59 As Brown puts this, building walls along borders actually reveals the weakness rather than the strength of states: "What appears at first blush as the articulation of state sovereignty actually expresses its diminution relative to other kids of state forces—the waning relevance and cohesiveness of the form" (*Walled States*, 24).

60 For example, Brown, *States of Injury*, 99.

INDEX

abortion, xii, 121, 169n18
absorption, 9, 34, 58
accumulation, 61, 93, 141;
hoarding, 65, 73; primitive, 7,
8; property, 37, 57, 146
Adams, Carol, 120–21, 122
Adorno, Theodor, 14
aesthetics, xxxii, 24, 29, 63, 136,
172n92; discourses of, xi, xii,
4, 43, 47; judgments based on,
44, 147
agency, 7, 49, 51, 148–49;
declining, 20, 39; digestive
subject and, 21, 63, 91;
humanist concept of, 129,
130, 131, 132; in obesity
debates, xxvi–xxvii; political,
xxviii, 40–41, 53, 152
agribusiness, 99, 112–13. *See also*
Big Food
agriculture, 35, 168n13; fuel use,
99–100, 108; globalization
of, xii, xiii; production
increases, x, xxiii, 73, 76, 93;
subsidies for, 76, 81, 111, 113;
urbanization's effects on,
xx–xxi. *See also* farmers and
farming; farmers' markets;

local foods movement;
organic foods movement
alienation, 16, 47; and
globalization, 103, 110; Hegel
on, 58; local foods movement
and, 100–103, 107–8; Marx on,
60, 68
America. *See* United States (U.S.)
American Obesity Association, 77
amphetamines, 11, 161n42
animals, 51, 53, 56, 125, 182n47;
domesticated, 124–25;
eating, 115, 139; humans'
relationship with, 27, 122,
123–27, 139, 140, 183n54;
killing of, xxxi, 123–24, 128,
133, 146–47, 151, 153–54,
181n40; not serving whole,
28, 164n13; rights of, xi–xii,
120, 123, 129, 183n39, 184n65;
suffering of, xvi, 121, 132;
treatment of, xiv, xviii, 101,
128, 139, 181n40, 182n36. *See
also* cows; horses; meat eating
and meat industry
anorexia nervosa, xvi, 12, 64, 85
anxieties, 12, 19, 30, 130, 145; over
bodily functions, 37, 43, 136;
over food, xiii, xxii, xxx–xxxi,

relationship to, 148, 149,
176n67
biosociality, 183n54
biotechnology, 98, 149, 153,
186n30; innovations in, xviii,
126, 141–42, 147
blood, drinking of, 116, 117,
180n5, 181n17
bodies, 51, 81, 143; body politic's
relationship to, 10, 11, 24–29,
94; controlling through diet,
78, 86, 110, 150; Descartes
on, 165n29, 170n40; energy
transactions in, 6, 8–9, 11,
41, 60, 108; equilibrium of,
56, 61–62; gendered, 7, 127;
governed by messages, 18,
20; Hobbes on, 39–40, 42, 44,
55; individual, 5, 52; integrity
of, xviii, 31, 44, 144–45;
knowledge of, 21, 83; Locke
on, xxxii, 52, 55; mechanized
views of, 3, 4, 5, 8, 10–11, 38;
mind over, 27, 29, 31–32, 34,
37, 164n25; as objects, 31–32,
136; orifices of, 27–28, 136;
privatizing functions of, xxi,
24–29, 43, 80, 137; scientific
understanding of, xvii, xxxii,
174n29; social, 5, 163n5;
social contract's relationship
to, 38–42, 131. See also
embodiment; human beings;
human-nonhuman border;
self-others border
body mass index (BMI), 74, 86,
173–74n18
body politic, xxviii, 28, 37, 38,
43–44, 48, 87, 130, 136, 148,
163n5, 166n53, 166n59;
bodies' relationship to, 10, 11,
24–29, 94; digestive turn in

political thought and, 47–49,
55–66; transition to social
contract from, 24, 42, 43–44,
90. See also politics
Bookchin, Murray, 93
borders, 130, 151, 164n22; anxiety
over, 30, 99; changing
understandings of, 102–3;
national, xxii, xxiii, 84, 135,
148, 150, 188n59. See also
human-nonhuman border;
public-private border;
self-other border; self-world
border; species: borders
between; subject-object
border
border security, xiii, xxii, xxiii, 84,
100, 116, 148, 151; obesity
and, xxvi, 72, 74, 86, 87,
88, 90
Bordo, Susan, 6–7, 29–32, 34, 36,
63, 123
boycotts, xiv, 109, 128
breeding, 126, 164n13. See also
meat eating and meat
industry
Brillat-Savarin, Jean Anthelme, 78,
80–81, 165n26
Brown, Wendy, xxiii–xxiv, 112,
155–56n11, 169n27
Brownell, Kelly, xiii, xxvi, 75, 77,
79, 89
Bruch, Hilde, 20, 85; *Eating
Disorders*, 12
Büchner, Ludwig, 54, 55, 63, 65,
67; *Kraft und Stoff (Force and
Matter)*, 53, 61
bulimia, 12, 85
Bulliet, Richard, xx, 101, 123, 127,
164n13
bureaucracy, 29–30, 43, 66
burping, 28, 80

commodities, 15, 60–61, 62, 171n71
communication, 43, 87; technologies of, 15–16, 102, 130, 147, 149, 153. *See also* information
communism, 62–63, 129, 145. *See also* socialism
communitarianism, xvii, 56, 136
communities, xix, 23, 145, 153; gated, xiii, 148; local foods movement's building of, xix, xxxi, 100–104; ownership by, 111–12. *See also* collective living
Community Supported Agriculture (CSA), 106, 110, 111–12. *See also* local foods movement
Comte, Auguste, 55
Connolly, William, xvii, xxv, 32, 66, 138, 160n24, 187n39
consciousness, 25, 34, 35, 43, 58, 165n43
constipation, 58, 64
constitutionalism, xxviii, 52, 60, 163n5, 168n1
consumerism and consumers, 13, 20, 105, 160n24, 188n57; benevolent, 111–12; choices made by, 73, 82, 94, 112, 135; citizenship and, xxiii, 106, 108, 109, 178–79n41; politics of, xxiii–xxiv, 94, 109–10, 113, 127, 150; producers building relationships with, 100–101, 103, 107, 108, 109, 111; responsible, xiv, xxii, xxiii, xxvii, 73, 110
consumption, x, 8, 15, 151, 153; ethics in, 93–94; Marx on, 60–61; of material objects, 58–59;

as metaphor, xvii, 169n29; politics of, xxiii–xxiv, 105, 106–7, 111, 113, 135; productive, 62, 108; public acts of, xxx, 27–28; responsible, 90, 111, 135
contagion. *See* disease(s); obesity: as epidemic
contamination, 35, 37, 98, 106, 137, 140, 143–44, 147. *See also* dirt: American obsession with
contracts, 38–42, 56, 63, 94, 113, 131; Hegel on, 55, 170n37; metaphor of, 26, 38, 44, 130, 170n37. *See also* social contract(s)
control, 110, 112, 147, 151. *See also* regulation; self-control
Coole, Diana, *New Materialisms*, xvii
Copernican Revolution, 3–4, 17
corporations, xxiv, 79, 172n89; power of, 14, 71, 75–76. *See also* Big Food; Big Organic; *and individual corporations*
Council on Bioethics, 142
counterculture movement, 1960s, 95, 96–97, 110
Coveney, John, 3
cows, 105, 141, 183n54; eating, xv, xviii, 116
Craig, Geoffrey, 100, 177n13
creationism, 49
criminal justice system. *See* justice
Critser, Greg, xiii, 14, 76, 81, 174n34
Cruikshank, Barbara, 6, 20
CSA. *See* Community Supported Agriculture (CSA)
cuisine, x, xxi, 96; national, xxvii, 17, 72, 89, 100
Cullather, Nick, 178n18

of, xviii, 48; disgust over, xxi, 139; European medical discoveries regarding, 50–51; metaphor of, xvii, xxv, xxxii, 56, 58–60, 66, 93, 169n29

digestive subjectivity, ix–x, 63, 66–69, 149–54; politics and, xvi, xxix, xxxiii; reimagining, 131, 136, 148; use of term, xvii, xviii

digestive turn, 1, 44–45, 47–69, 129, 131, 148–49, 151–52; American approach to food, 67–69; anxieties associated with, 71–72; body politic and, 47–49, 55–66; German origins of, 66–67; Hegel's, xxxii, 55–60, 63–65, 68, 93, 170n36; liberal, 135, 136, 145, 147; Marx's, xxxii, 56, 60–64, 68, 93, 144; metaphors of, 43; Nietzsche's, xxix–xxx, xxxii, 63, 64–66, 68, 93

dinitrophenol, 9, 11, 160n34

Dionne, E. J., 184n1

dirt, American obsession with, xxx, 43, 95–96, 97, 185n11. See also contamination

disability, 116, 141, 143, 144

disease(s), 77, 91, 139; of civilization, xxv, 89; immigration and, 84–85; obesity seen as, 71, 77, 82–87, 88, 90, 135, 175n39; rhetoric of, 83, 84, 88, 175n39

disgust: associated with killing animals, 123–24; over bodily functions, xxi, 25, 28, 59, 139, 187n39; definitions of, 137, 185n6; with democratic

process, xxxiii, 135–54; digestive subjectivity and, 149–54; discourse of, 132, 139, 143, 147; over politics, 96, 103, 140–49, 184n1

disorder(s): bodily, 43, 175n39; digestive, 50, 64; eating, 6, 11, 12, 68, 85, 161n46; political, 43; social, xxx

diuretics, 9, 11

Douglas, Mary, xxx, 43, 80, 88, 96, 99, 119, 138, 144, 185n11

drinking, 7, 27. See also blood: drinking of

drugs. See dietary-pharmaceutical complex

dualism: Cartesian, 39, 41, 50, 66, 80–81; Locke's, 34, 38

eating: as agricultural act, xi, 93; of animals, xv, xviii, 115, 116, 117, 139, 180n5; culture of, xxvii–xxviii; Hobbes on, 37–42; human being's relationship to, xii, xv–xvi, 1, 62, 63, 64; labor and, 57–58; Locke on, 33, 36, 37; Nietzsche on, xv–xvi, xxix–xxx; ontopolitics of, 29–32; politics of, xix, 24–29, 93–113; privatization of, xxi, 23–45; prohibited items, 116, 117, 119; in public, xix–xx, 24, 37, 45, 142, 187n33; reflections on, xxviii, 153; rituals of, xv, xix, 23, 45. See also appetite; assimilation; food; meat eating and meat industry; overeating

eating disorders, 6, 11, 12, 68, 85, 161n46

E. coli, 68, 71, 97

ecology, xi, 45, 66, 113, 129, 133

economics and economy, xvi, 2,
6, 63, 78, 141, 153; bodily,
61–62; bourgeois, 29, 32, 64;
capitalist, xxiii, 5, 51; dieting
and, 5, 13; discourses of, 6,
47, 54, 55; of food, 8–9, 47,
93; global, xv, xxiv, 87–88;
industrial, 15, 18, 62; local
food, 101, 103–4; market,
21, 63, 146; Marx on, 9,
48, 60, 64; obesity and, 74,
77–78, 159n18; privatization
of, 5, 25; service, 15, 18;
transformations in, xx–xxi,
76; U.S., 2, 95. *See also* capital
and capitalism; consumerism
and consumers
Elias, Norbert: on civilizing
process, 26–28, 30, 35, 37,
42, 56, 80, 146, 164n13; on
manners, 26, 32, 80, 137, 140,
142
elitism, 68, 148, 178n34
embodiment, xv, 41, 165n43. *See
also* bodies
embryonic stem cell research,
xviii, 142
empowerment, 12, 14, 20, 21, 110,
115, 160n24
energy: agricultural use of, 99–100,
108; conservation of, 49–50,
55, 63, 65; conversion of,
51, 62; food, 56, 61; human,
53–54, 61, 63, 171n69;
transactions of, 6, 8–9, 11, 41,
60, 108. *See also* calories
England, 54, 84, 123, 166n53
Enlightenment, the, 3, 102, 121,
123
entitlement, xxviii, 17, 21
entropy, 11, 49, 99
environment, the, 79, 110,

115–16, 184n70; individuals'
transacting with, 35–36, 56,
64, 145. *See also* nature
epidemiology, xxvi, 84–85, 86,
87, 90, 130, 158n47. *See also*
obesity: as epidemic
epistemology, xviii, xxviii, 24,
29–32, 47, 63
equality, 53, 90–91, 94, 129. *See
also* inequality
Esposito, Roberto, 42, 145, 148
ethical turn, 127–29, 148–49,
151–52, 187–88n50; liberal,
135, 136, 145; posthumanist,
131, 132
ethics, xviii, 41–42, 65–66, 103,
112; discourses of, xi, xii, xvi,
4, 55; food-related issues, xix,
xxviii, 93–94; market-related,
106, 152; of meat eating,
xxx, xxxi, 115, 116, 121, 123,
126, 127–29; Protestant, 4,
159n18; of vegetarianism,
101, 127–29. *See also*
bioethics
European Union (EU), xxii, 100
evolution, 49, 55, 126
exchange, 48, 54, 61; capitalist, 30,
32, 61, 62, 63, 65; of matter,
52, 54, 57
excretion, 51, 55, 58; disgust over,
28, 59, 139; sites of, 27, 47. *See
also* defecation; feces
exercise, xiv, 7, 8, 10
externalization, 57–58, 62

family meals, decline in, xix–xx,
xxii, 23, 68
fantasy, 15, 72, 103; of sovereignty,
65–66, 69
Farm Bill Extension Act of 2007,
111, 113

farmers and farming, 104, 110, 124, 179n51; backyard, xii, xiv, 106; family, 97, 106–7, 108. *See also* agriculture; organic foods movement

farmers' markets, xi, xiv, 106, 110, 153; community-building through, xix, xxxi, 100–104. *See also* local foods movement

fast food, xix, xxi, 23, 68, 107, 172–73n3, 178n34

fat: dietary, xiii, 17, 18, 51, 89, 162n72; meaning of, 72–77, 82–83, 89. *See also* obesity

fat acceptance movement, 82, 150, 160n26, 175n37

fatigue, 8, 11, 13

fear, xiii, 13, 35, 67–68, 137. *See also* anxieties

feces, xxxiii, 26, 35, 59, 137–38. *See also* defecation; excretion

feminism and feminists, xvii, xx, 31, 56; on diet, 12, 19, 77, 82; on meat industry, 120–21; philosophies of, 127, 137

fertilizers, 73, 94, 168n13, 177n8

festivals, eating at, xv, xix, 23, 27–28, 45

fetishes and fetishism, xiii, 63, 65, 125, 139, 171n71, 185–86n19

Feuerbach, Ludwig, 52, 53, 67, 145, 165n26, 169n17

Feyerabend, Paul, 159n8

Fight Club (film, Fincher), 160n24

finance. *See* economics and economy

Fisher, Irving, *How to Live*, 8–10

Fisk, Eugene Lyman, *How to Live*, 8–10

fitness, physical. *See* exercise

Fitzhugh, George, *Cannibals All!*, 117

Flathman, Richard, 44

Flegal, Katherine, 83

Fletcher, Horace, 9

Foer, Jonathan Safran, 122, 126, 184n70; *Eating Animals*, 128

food, 36, 51, 52, 76, 105, 137; anxieties over, xiii, xxii, xxx–xxxi, 44, 67–68, 71–72, 150; choices of, xi, xix–xxiv, xxiii, 18, 108–11, 178–79n41; contamination concerns, xxvi, 35, 95–96, 106; culture of, xi, xv, xix, xxvii–xxviii, 20, 23; debates over, 48, 71, 147; democratic ethos of, xxiv, 94, 153; economy of, 8–9, 47, 93; energy from, 56, 61; guilt over, 147, 164n16; immediate, 97–98, 100–101, 110; industrialization of, 23–24, 96, 98, 99, 108, 113; literature on, xxv–xxvi, xxvii, 153, 164n16; low-carb, 17, 18; packaged, xix–xxi, 13, 23, 68, 76, 139, 154; pathological relationship to, 77–78, 81, 85; privatization of, xix–xxiv, 44, 103, 106, 136; production of, 10, 98, 99, 100–103, 108, 123–24; protein-based, xxi, 17, 18, 19; responsible, xiv, xxv, 93–94, 98, 100–101, 106; ritual consumption of, xv, xix, 23, 45; scholarship on, xxvii–xxxi; seventeenth-century transitions in, 23–45; in U.S., xiv, 44–45, 67–69, 93, 98, 105–6, 120, 178–79n41; in worldviews, ix–x, xxi, xxxiii–xxxiv. *See also* dairy industry; diet; eating; fast food; meat eating and meat industry; nutrition

Food, Inc. (film, Kenner), xiii

governance, xviii, 100, 130, 149, 150, 153–54; democratic, xxviii, 105. *See also* self-governance

government, xiii, 106, 146, 163n5; representative, xiv, xvii, 32–33, 38, 105, 132–33, 135, 145. *See also* constitutionalism; democracy

Gregory, Frederick, 53, 169n17

Grosz, Elizabeth, 31–32, 34, 35, 59, 123, 140

guilt: associated with killing animals, 123–24, 139; over food, 147, 164n16; postdomestic, 101–2

Guthman, Julie, 95, 101, 106, 107–8, 111

Haber, Fritz, 177n8

Hale, David, 25, 38, 166n53

Halweil, Brian, 100–101, 103, 105, 106

Haraway, Donna, 122, 124, 128, 148, 149; on companion species, 125–27, 182n54

Hardt, Michael, 87, 100, 130

Harvey, Arthur, 179n46

Harvey, David, 15, 102, 155–56n11

health, 8, 78; obesity's effects on, 82–87; threats to, 10, 11, 13, 96–97. *See also* public health

health-industrial complex, xxv, 77, 89

heart disease, 8, 12, 68, 83

Hegel, Georg Wilhelm Friedrich, 54, 148, 152, 153; on alienation, 47, 58; *Aufhebung*, 57; on consumption, 169n29; on contract theory, 55, 170n37; on desire for recognition, 145–46; dialectics of, 48, 56, 57, 58–59, 66–67; digestive turn in, xxxii, 55–60, 63–65, 68, 93, 170n36; *Logic*, 56; *Phenomenology of Spirit*, 56, 57; *Philosophy of Nature*, 56, 59; politics of, 66–69; subjectivity in, 48, 57, 136

Helmholtz, Hermann von, 55, 168n6

Heyes, Cressida, 5–6, 14, 20

high-fructose corn syrup, xiii, 71, 76, 85

Hirsch, Jules, 173n12

Hobbes, Thomas, xxxii, 55, 137, 167n70; contract theory of, 145, 146; *De Corpore*, 39, 42, 166n53; on individual sovereignty, 49, 80, 166–67n66; *Leviathan*, xxviii, xxix, 24, 38, 44, 151, 166n53; on liberalism, xxi, 37–42, 44, 166n53; materialism of, 38, 39, 40–41, 42; metaphysics in, 38, 41; politics of, 37–42

Holocaust, 13–14, 118, 177n8

homosexuality, 143, 187n44. *See also* sex and sexuality

Hoover, Herbert, 9, 160n32

hormonal paradigm of dieting, xxxi, 14–17, 18, 19, 88, 162n76

horses, 183n47; as meat, 116, 117, 180n5

human beings, xviii, 24, 130, 149; animals' relationship with, 27, 122, 123–27, 139, 140, 183n54; eating and, xii, xv–xvi, 1, 62, 63, 64; energy in, 53–54, 61, 63, 171n69; engagement with the world, x–xi, 47, 57–58, 64, 66, 68–69; exceptionalism of, 119, 137; nature's relationship to, 66, 101, 125, 131, 159n19;

communication; data collection and management; knowledge

ingestion, 27, 37, 40, 51, 61–62, 139

institutions, xiii, 42, 149, 150; loss of faith in, xxv, 88, 89–91, 103, 106–7, 154

internalization, xv, 30, 57–58, 62, 64

Internet, the, 15, 18, 110

Jameson, Fredric, 15, 91

Jay, Martin, 66–67, 164n22, 172n92

Jeffersonian ideals, 103, 110

Jenny Craig weight loss program, 6, 14

John of Salisbury, 25

Johnson, Mark, xvii, xxviii

Joliffe, Norman, diet developed by, 12, 18

justice, xiii, 57, 59, 95, 172n96

Kant, Immanuel, 57, 131, 165n29, 169n28; dualism of, 50; idealism in, 65

Kass, Leon, xvii, 186n31, 187n33; on cannibalism, 118, 119, 142, 169n18; on vegetarianism, 121, 122, 125, 127; on "you are what you eat," xv, xvi, xxx

Kellogg, John Harvey, 9–10, 19, 64

Kellogg, William, 10

Keynes, John Maynard, 7–8, 13, 16

Kingsolver, Barbara, xi, 97, 103, 104–5, 147, 151

Kirkland, Anna, 141

Klosterman, Chuck, 72, 80, 90, 173n4

knowledge, ix, xiii–xiv, xxviii, 5, 29, 33, 42, 66. See also information

Kojève, Alexandre, 62, 66, 170n36; on Hegel, 57–58, 59, 67

Kolata, Gina, 173n12

Korsmeyer, Carolyn, 165n29

Kraftwechsel. See energy: conversion of

Kristeva, Julia, 138–39

Kuhn, Thomas, 2–4, 16, 50, 55, 63, 159n8

Kymlicka, Will, 59

labor, xvi, 6, 16, 63, 105, 179n44; eating and, 57–58; exploitation of, xiv, 107–8, 110, 171n71; Locke on, 35–37; Marx on, 60, 62, 117, 159n19, 162, 170n36, 171n69. *See also* farmers and farming; industrialization; producers and production

Lacan, Jacques, 67

Lakoff, George, xvii, xxviii

land: allocation of, x, xi, xxiv; cultivation of, 107, 179n51; enclosure of, xxi, 24, 30; ownership of, 104, 105, 108, 111; relationship to, 93, 95–96, 100–103, 106

Lappe, Frances Moore, *Diet for a Small Planet*, 94

Latour, Bruno, xvii, 87, 130, 147

learning, xxix–xxx, 64. *See also* knowledge

Lebesco, Kathleen, 75, 80, 141, 159n18; *Revolting Bodies*, 82

Lefort, Claude, 163n5

legality, xvii, xxv, 26, 55, 90–91

Lestringant, Frank, 117, 118

Levenstein, Harvey, xxvii, 179n42

Lévi-Strauss, Claude, 43

liberalism, xxi, 5, 10, 24–25, 44, 60, 69, 104, 116, 135, 140, 167n70, 169n27, 176n67;

nineteenth-century, 51–54; scientific, 48, 53, 68, 121, 148

matter, 2, 4, 41; conversion of, 51, 62; eternality of, 53; exchange of, 52, 54, 57

McCarthy, Cormac, *The Road*, 117

McDonald's restaurants, 68, 72–73, 81, 97, 172n2

McKibben, Bill, 97, 98–99, 101, 103

McWilliams, James, 178–79n41

meat eating and meat industry, 115–33; butchering, 164n13; cannibalism and, 117–23; discourses of, 132, 135; disgust regarding, 139–40, 141, 142; environmental concerns regarding, 115–16, 120; ethics related to, xxx, xxxi, 115–16, 121, 123, 126, 127–29; feminist views of, 120–21; industrialization of, 115–16, 184n69; livestock raising, 126, 184n65; postdomesticity and, 123–27; posthuman democracy and, 129–33. *See also* cows; horses; hunting

mechanization. *See* industrialization; thermodynamics

media, 14, 20, 99, 113

medicine, 8, 19, 49, 50–51, 179n42

memory, 34, 64

men, 7, 160n24, 186n27

Mendelsohn, Everett, 50

metabolic paradigm of dieting, 8–11, 13, 16, 18, 150

metabolism, 62, 146; of bodies, 25, 26; body weight as function of, 4, 85; Marx's metabolic rift, xvi, xxviii, 96, 99, 101, 108,

151; processes of, 27, 44, 139; thermodynamics and, 60, 108

metaphors: of body politic, 43–44, 130, 166n53; of consumption, xvii, 169n29; contract, 26, 38, 44, 130, 170n37; of dieting, 10–11; food as, xvi, xxix–xxx; network, 87, 130–31, 151; ocular, 66–67; political, xxviii, 24, 48; structural, xvii, xxviii. *See also* digestion: metaphor of

metaphysics, 50; Hobbes's use of, 38, 41

Metropolitan Life Insurance Company, 74

Middle Ages, 43, 65; bodily functions during, 26–28, 44; transition to modern era, 24, 25, 30, 130

Midgley, Mary, 186n30

Milgram, Stanley, conformity studies, 14

Millan, Cesar, 125

Miller, William Ian, *The Anatomy of Disgust*, 137–40, 146, 185n6, 185n11

mind, the, 39; over body, 27, 29, 31–32, 34, 37, 164n25; Locke on, 165n43; Nietzsche on, 65

Mitchell, W. J. T., 123, 182n39

modernism, 13, 64. *See also* postmodernism; premodernism

Moleschott, Jakob, 54, 55, 61, 65, 144, 145; *Der Kreislauf des Lebens (The Cycle of Life)*, 53; *Die Lehre der Nahrungsmittel: Für das Volk (The Theory of Food: For the People)*, 52, 67, 169n17; *Die Physiologie der Nahrungsmittel (The Physiology of Food)*, 52

discourses of, 103, 114, 135, 144, 147, 153, 159n18; as disease, 71, 77, 82–87, 88, 90, 135, 175n39; as epidemic, xiv, xxvi, xxviii, 72–73, 81, 90–91, 144, 162n72, 174n23, 176n53; genetic factors, 4, 85; globalization's relationship to, 87–88, 150; health risks of, 10, 74; lies associated with, 87–91; meaning of, 72–77, 82–83, 89; moral judgments regarding, 10, 13, 22, 82, 90, 93, 141, 159n11; politics of, xxiii, 73, 75–78, 82, 87, 88, 144; poverty and, 73, 81; rates of, xxvi, 68, 73, 75–78, 83–84, 86, 91, 174n22; responsibility for, xx, xxvi–xxvii, 4, 72–82, 83, 87–88, 90, 93, 150, 174n34. *See also* dieting; overeating

objectivity, xxii, 29–30, 44, 47, 66; crisis of, xvii, xviii, 131, 147

OFPA. *See* Organic Foods Production Act (OFPA) of 1990

oil, x, 94, 98–99, 108, 178n18

Oliver, J. Eric, 83, 89, 174n23, 176n53; *Fat Politics*, 77, 88

ontology, xvii–xviii, xxvii, 32; of identity and, xvii, 53; liberal, 140, 145; Locke's, xxix

ontopolitics, 119, 129; definition of, xvii; of individual sovereignty, 33, 40, 41, 44, 80, 90; liberal, 49, 51, 63, 67–69, 85–86, 93, 103, 112, 135–36, 139, 147, 152–53; of liberalism, xxxii, 29–32, 33, 37, 39, 43–44, 136, 150; network, 130–31; of representative government, 91, 132–33, 145, 148; social

contract and, 48, 52, 54, 144; vocabulary of, xxxi, 130

Orbach, Susie, *Fat Is a Feminist Issue*, 12, 20, 82

organic foods movement, 93, 108; labeling of, xiii, 105–6; shift to local foods movement, 94–100; sociability and, 101, 103; trust in, 106–7, 148, 179n42. *See also* Big Food; local foods movement

Organic Foods Production Act (OFPA) of 1990, 96, 103, 105–6

organ transplants, 180n5

Orlie, Melissa, 65–66

Orwell, George, *1984*, 13

Ostherr, Kirsten, 86

otherness and others, xxxiii, 127, 146; ethical commitment to, 127, 131; internalization of, 58, 62. *See also* self-others border

outside-inside border, xxx, 42, 64. *See also* self-world border

overeating, ix, 10, 14, 15, 73

oxygen, 8, 51, 52

pain, 31, 137. *See also* suffering

paradigm shifts, 47–48, 50, 51, 145, 159n8

Parkins, Wendy, 100, 177n13

Patel, Raj, *Stuffed and Starved*, xiii

People for the Ethical Treatment of Animals (PETA), 182n40

People's Park (Berkeley), 95

Personal Responsibility in Food Consumption Act of 2003, xxii, xxvi, 72, 79, 150

pesticides, 94, 96, 98, 106, 177n8

PETA. *See* People for the Ethical Treatment of Animals (PETA)

Peters, Lulu Hunt, *Diet and Health*, 9, 10

Rajan, Tilottama, 58
rationality, xxiii, 32, 52, 107, 132, 169n28. *See also* reason
Rawls, John, 33
Rawson, Claude, 118
reason, 30–31, 38, 121, 130, 144, 148, 151. *See also* rationality
recognition, 67, 82, 145–46; politics of, 59, 66, 187n38
Regan, Tom, 120, 122, 128, 132
regulation, xiii, 1, 19, 75, 109, 129. *See also* control; self-control
religion(s), xxi, 3, 16, 30, 38, 65, 117; food in rituals of, xv, xix, 23, 45
representation, xviii, 68, 135, 151; democratic, xiii, 131, 132, 146; narratives of, xxxiii, 67; political, xxv, 32, 54, 66, 115, 164n22. *See also* government: representative
respiration, 33, 40, 51
responsibility, xii, xiv, xxviii, xxxiii, 42, 63, 65, 86, 130, 135, 148, 153; decline in, 71, 116; food-related, xiv, xxv, 1, 44–45, 93–94, 98, 100–101, 106; identity and, xviii, 66; ideology of, xxii, xxxiii, 36, 81, 119, 135, 153; liberal rhetorics of, 82, 94; Lockean approach to, 79–80; narratives of, xiii, xxxiii, 25; for obesity, xx, xxvi–xxvii, 4, 14, 15, 72–82, 83, 87–88, 90, 93, 150, 174n34; ontopolitics of, 45, 132–33; politics of, x, 20–21, 47, 90, 112, 131, 151–52; in *Super Size Me*, 172–73n3; threats to, xvii, 149. *See also* consumerism and consumers: responsible
responsible foods movement.
See food: responsible; food activism; local foods movement; organic foods movement
ressentiment, xvi, 47, 64, 65, 101–2
restaurants, xix, 95–96. *See also* McDonald's restaurants
revolutions of 1848, 50, 54, 67
Riesman, David, *The Lonely Crowd*, 14
rights, xi, xiii, 115; animal, xi–xii, 120, 123, 129, 182n39, 184n65; discourses on, 68, 112, 145; human, 132–33, 152; liberal, 43, 56; property, xiv, 54, 100, 105
Rinella, Steven, 124, 177n11
Robbins, John, *Diet for a New America*, 181n23
Robin, Corey, 13
Robin Hood Commission, 95
Romero, George, 117
Rose, Nikolas, 86
Rozin, Paul, 137, 142
Rubner, Max, 51, 61

Salatin, Joel, 179n46, 179n51
saliva, 26, 28, 137–38
salmonella, xiii, 68
Schaffer, Michael, 124
Schlosser, Eric, xi, 76, 188n57; *Fast Food Nation*, 72–73, 124
Schwartz, Hillel, 7–9, 10, 13, 17, 82–83, 160n26
science, xiii, xvii, 44, 67, 106, 136; bourgeois, 29, 66; dietary, xxxii, 51; discourses of, xii, 43, 44, 47, 54; history of, 2–4, 16, 55; materialist, 121, 148; modern, xxix, 42, 45, 100; politics and, 50, 159n8
segregation, 103–4

CHAD LAVIN is an associate professor in the Department of Political Science and the Alliance for Social, Political, Ethical, and Cultural Thought (ASPECT) at Virginia Tech. He has previously published *The Politics of Responsibility* and essays in social and political theory.